ENERGIZING SELF-TRUST:

7 Steps for Reclaiming Your Power

By

J Lawrence Maerz BA

Published in the United States by
Emotional Troubleshooter, LLC
ISBN 978-0986436451
Library of Congress: 2015932044

*This book is dedicated to Dani, Jessica, Kristie, John,
Marilyn, Rosa & Shannon at Word-of-Mouth
in Sarasota who gave my visits special
attention and made me feel like family.*

*Special thanks goes to Kala Ambrose who marketing
wisdom and advice have proven invaluable.*

*"Until you've been washed ashore, you can't know
how all encompassing the sea has become…"*

-J Lawrence Maerz

ENERGIZING SELF-TRUST

7 STEPS FOR RECLAIMING YOUR POWER

When I started writing this book I was primarily focused solely on what I was reacting to as I examined my own motivations. But the more I read and the more I observed the world around me in terms of what only I understood, I began to see a pattern emerge that told me that there is a rudimentary structuring of our personalities that takes place based on our Western European culture's childrearing practices underlying all of us and forming the basis for the reasons why and if we do what we choose to do. The problem now becomes how do all of us express it?

In our social society we have many different perspectives from which to observe and assess our lives. We have scientists, philosophers, economists, doctors, lawyers, biologists and a whole host of other professionals and laymen all with their own language as to how they describe what they know and observe. So the question for me that begged to be answered was How do I present to others what I've come to understand and used myself so that the widest sampling of our society might gain a clear understanding of it, free of the petty, professionally structured idiosyncrasies that create annoying difficulties for us in understanding concepts while operating "on the same page"? And then I remembered a discovery in the field of anthropology - the Rosetta Stone. It describes the same scripture in three distinctly different languages allowing scientists to make startling breakthroughs in understanding the continuity existing between sequentially different cultures. Then it occurred to me: Why not write the same book from different perspectives or languages so everyone can operate on, essentially, the same page when learning to understand and program motivation? What a beautiful concept.

In this light it became necessary to look at how our minds develop, but not only from a psychological perspective, which is the point of view that is most often presented. This was not enough; most people get lost in the theory and jargon. A second perspective became necessary. For the ordinary person, you and me as the layman, to understand the origins and dynamics of *Self-Trust* and motivation the explanation had to come from building a recognizable process of development, as perceived from our childhood perspective without all the jargon and seemingly ambiguous and confusing terms used in the professional and academic fields.

So here it is, my motivational Rosetta Stone. I've laid it out in three sections: a simple progression of seven steps and an explanation of what is happening in two languages - for the layman and the therapist. Hopefully, this will help us cross traditional barriers into a common understanding.

All three sections may be read and understood independent of each other but I recommend that you read them in order, as the continuity will yield more depth and, from a selfish perspective, will give you a better handle on the thought processes I went through in setting it up this way.

Introduction

As far back as I can consciously remember and up until the last few years my life has been a series of continuous and cascading reactions. My attention was always on what was occurring outside of my private internal world which I felt was the only world that I was able to participate in and perceive. I was hypnotized by its beauty but deathly afraid of its danger. Notice, I didn't say understand. Until recently, I never did.

Like a turtle sensing danger outside his shell, I felt my only refuge for safety from the constant assault of emotional triggering was to pull within. So I did. I became an introvert. Through my upbringing I learned to be afraid of everything that happened outside my shell. I believed that it threatened to consume my very energy and 'being' piece by piece, and if I remained outside my shell for any length of time, there would shortly be nothing left of me. To live, I had to occasionally go outside looking for food and nurturance. I darted out, gathering what I needed, and scurried back in like a squirrel. I lived my life fearing to attract the attention of those outside lest I be gobbled up by those much stronger and more powerful than I. When I went back inside, some of them even attacked my shell attempting to force me out so I could become their dinner. This made me all the more fearful and to hide inside all the more tightly. But as I grew, a curious thing happened. Trapped inside my shell, I began to look around. I began to notice all my past experiences piled in a dark corner and hidden from the light. I began to dig into that pile. And dig, and dig and dig. I became obsessed with finding what was at the bottom of that pile that held everything so tightly in this dark corner. This obsession became my path, my life, my reason for being. The number one question on my mind became, "How and why have I come to live this way?"

I liken my life to a movie I saw many years ago called Journey to the Center of the Earth. Oh, not the sensationalized one from 2008 with Brendon Frasier chasing and protecting the little boy from all the prehistoric monsters wanting to gobble him up. That was fun to watch but a major departure from the message the earlier 1959 movie with Pat Boone and James Mason had planted in my mind. No, the earlier movie was about going deeper and deeper inside the volcano to find the origins and ancestors of what lay outside the cone on the surface; to find the history and the civilization that had begun it all. Following them I felt the pressure as they crept through passageways that were getting narrower and narrower until they finally broke through into a tremendous internal cavern - a whole different world. There they found oceans to cross with voracious monsters lurking beneath the surface waiting to consume them and tremendous prehistoric land beasts fighting among themselves and threatening to crush them as they rolled in combat. And then, after finding an earlier explorer and the remains of the previous civilization, the volcano erupted spewing its hot emotional current out from its core, landing them back in the daylight of the surface with an understanding of where they had been, what they had found and, what it meant.   How close is this analogy to what we find inside of us, to the things we have buried and forgotten but that yet hold such influence over how we face the outside world? How can we ever hope to feel peace within with the constant gnawing of unidentified and unclarified emotional currents coursing through our lives leaving us only to helplessly react whenever they are triggered? What will it take to make us turn inward and look at where these triggers were formed and why we have become so accustomed to reacting to them the way we do?

Each one of us has to arrive at our own limit of what we are able to endure before we cry uncle and give in to what needs to be done. Even Popeye arrives at a place where he says, "I took all I can stands and I can't stands no more!" and then whirls into action. Will it take becoming totally immobilized by fear and depression before we come to the realization that it is necessary for our growth to trust ourselves or will we continue to submit to being strangled by the petrified forest of "traditional" roots and vines that have choked the fight out of us since childhood? Some of us go to our graves this way never knowing or believing there was a different way. Many of us arrive at midlife and recognize that something has been missing and begin an inward journey eventually erupting out through the top of our volcano. Some of us recognize and accept the hopelessness of our situation and slide into endless depression. Some of us are fortunate enough to recognize the collapse of our *Self-Trust* and *Confidence* and embark on a courageous battle that regains the control of our lives. Some of us never even realize what is happening and just instinctively strike out blindly for freedom of expression, meeting insurmountable resistance. Whatever your reason or method of arrival toward picking up my book and questioning why your life is the way it is, I commend you. You have begun a journey that will take you to a place which will allow you total access to the energy and motivation that will bring you peace, tranquility and excitement about life again through regaining your *Self-Trust* and *Confidence* in who you are becoming and your right to do so.

OUR PATH TO EMPOWERMENT:

How Do We Get There?

The Childhood Landscape

We have spent many years building the emotional inertia that has led to our arrival at the place where we find ourselves now. We all feel that there were pivotal points in our lives where, if we had gone another way, we might not be where we are now. We usually see those experiences as choices we *had* to make based on our life circumstances. But those choices had *everything* to do with how we felt about ourselves at the time. And how we felt about ourselves at the time had everything to do with the way we were taught about how the world perceived us; more appropriately, how it perceived our value and worth as a person. We are still much the same, seeing those circumstances as the reason we are where we are at present. The underlying point is that we have allowed our value and worth to be determined by people *outside* of ourselves, continuing the training we received in childhood. That childhood training consisted of our parents indoctrinating us with the belief that they, as adults, knew better than we and that we must follow their given rules if we were to remain safe and in their good graces. We can understand how and why providing for our safety was necessary, for the most part, at that age, since we *didn't* know better and we *needed* their rules and guidance to keep us safe. However, an added benefit for our parents was that, in our following their rules, they had a means of controlling and directing not only our actions but our emotional responses. In this, the extent of their need to do so depended very much on *their* emotional experience and maturity.

We still see ourselves now much the same way we believed the world saw us then, except that now it has a long history of reinforcement throughout repeating the same beliefs and patterns we were taught, over and over. Though we have mostly matured enough to physically see to our own safety, our emotional rapport with our parents still remains mostly intact as it was in our childhood. In terms of feeling a sense of belonging and connection with them, this may be seen as a positive quality, if that is our need or goal. But in venturing into the world, looking to manifest our own accomplishments, our rapport with them may present itself as an inhibition for us through being limited to handling life in the same ways our parents have indoctrinated us with and reflecting their methods.

The way the world sees and responds to us is deeply rooted in our opinions of ourselves. This is our personal inertia. Newton says that a thing that is moving will continue to move in the same direction and speed until something acts upon it to change both. He asserted that this is true for all earthly matter. What Newton couldn't know then, or maybe he did but just didn't say, was how right this was concerning *every* aspect of our lives. The law is also true for feelings, thoughts and their resultant emotions. So, if the forces acting on us are consistent, why would we change? If our social interaction remains consistent, why would we behave differently?

The way the world values us and our acceptance of it, is well integrated within our psyches. It could almost be compared to a systemic infection permeating the body and the only way to eliminate it is to kill the host it survives on. I'm painting a drastic picture, but I'm making a point about how deep and integral our social programming has been. There is almost no corner of our being where it has not penetrated. Notice I said *almost*. That "almost" corner, whether a conscious space or not, is available and is the place we need to work.

If you will, imagine we are in a thick forest wanting to clear some space where we might grow some food for nourishment. All we have is a pick, a saw and a shovel and the desire to create our own space. There are tremendous trees soaring overhead. There are smaller trees, brush, vines and undergrowth, all with intermingling and entangled roots that stretch into each other's space, strengthening their grip on each other, us and the land. When we look at the bigger picture, our task seems daunting and overwhelming. What are we to do? Simple. Dig where we stand. Make a space. Chop away the plants and the roots where we are standing. Work with what we can see and what we can expose in our small space. Pull it away and expose the fertile ground beneath our feet. Some roots and plants will come out easily; others will be stubborn and take more time and effort. We must be patient and persistent with ourselves. This is our space that we are reclaiming. When we finally break through and pull away all that has been holding the soil beneath our feet, we can feel a sigh of relief and a sense of release as we feel the peace and ease in our newly cleared space. Now we rest.

Just having become free of the strangling effects of the forest is, in itself, a relief and a shock to our system. It's as if we are coming out of a long tunnel and being overwhelmed by the light as we emerge. We are delighted and even almost surprised that we have been able to clear such a safe and peaceful space for ourselves. Part of that feeling includes a sense that that space is somehow familiar to us, almost like we belong there. As we relish the feeling of having our own space and the peace and contentment it begins to provide for us, our attention, once again, turns to the forest surrounding us and a sinking feeling of guilt and undeservedness creeps into our awareness. We have taken something that the forest around us had claimed and held. Did we have the right to claim our own space? Was it really *ours* or did it really belong to the forest? Do *we* belong to the forest? When we were a seedling the forest protected us and nurtured us. What do we really owe the forest? How? What must we do or be? We feel torn between our own space and the surrounding forest. We feel doubt about who we are and what we have done.

In our social environment, like the forest, any cleared space will eventually be reclaimed as small vines, roots and seedlings slowly begin growing into our space attempting to reclaim what was originally theirs. But any tree first began as a seedling and slowly, slowly grows to dominate its own space in the forest and, eventually, provides shade and protection through its presence. We realize then that if we are to remain in the forest it will take constant vigilance and clearing if we are to maintain the clarity and peace that we have created surrounding our being. Then, we must provide protection and nurturance for *our* seedlings as we expand even further. And they, in turn, will reclaim space from *us*. This is the nature of cycle in the forest. If we are to remain, we must maintain our awareness and a balance in our relationship with her. But that requires being in two worlds at once; our own, in which we must maintain clarity, and the forest's, in which we must be careful not to overrun *its* space with *our* intentions and actions or allow it to overrun ours.

The analogy of the forest is simple. To feel our own space we must cut away enough of the outside influences to find our personal space. We don't have to do anything else with the forest; just give us enough space to move and expand a bit. It is only then that we can see clearly what we feel. And then, knowing what we feel, we can come to a clear understanding of who or what we must grow into in order to fulfill our intentions for being in the forest in the first place. As a seedling, the most difficult part is feeling and believing that the forest determines who and what we should grow into. The full grown trees appear to have dominance over the forest, but they too are simply a part of a larger whole. We, as seedlings must, at some point, become responsible and accountable for our *own* space and growth if we are to grow into soaring trees. Creating and maintaining a balance in our existence with others is a much harder task than simply striving for and maintaining dominance or living in a completely submissive and servile position. Both of those are easy. To create and maintain balance, though, we must pay attention to providing nurturance on two fronts: to our *own* space and to the space of the forest. This is what the mystics have called "Walking the Middle Path."

Alone time, or our own "quiet space" in the forest, is probably one of the most sought after yet undervalued commodities in our materialistic world. We give it lip service but don't understand the point of it. We struggle, trying to accumulate privacy in the world, but are so caught up in the frenzy of acquiring it that we forget to occasionally just sit back and relish what we have accomplished. Usually, during those needed free times, we find ourselves conspiring and planning our next conquest, all the while forgetting to use the space for what our inner self has been yearning for; time to contemplate, time to relish our own feelings. I call alone time a commodity because our Western culture has interpreted it as simply an acquisition in our daily endeavors while never truly allowing us to partake of its fullest beauty and advantage. This is the space we clear under our feet in the forest. A place to relax, breathe, let go and trust that our space is our own and that we can feel safe in it, believing that there is nothing that can interfere with knowing what we feel there. At the risk of getting too metaphysical, I will simply say that for all spiritual disciplines this is the space that is used for meditation. Suffice it to say, meditation is simply centering and reacquainting yourself with your own inner space, and I'll leave it at that. You can explore types and methods of meditation at your own leisure.

So, now we're grounded, rested and ready to see the ways in which we can establish an expanding place for nourishment. What's our next step? I could say that our task is to literally reclaim space in the forest by unwinding each branch of the vines spiraling up the trunks of "our" trees and choking the life out of us. Instinctively, this would be our objective, but that would eventually only lead to creating more of the "dominance in the forest" perspective, especially if we were to set it on automatic, which so many of our promoted Western approaches have done. But I would like to return to "we must pay attention to providing nurturance on two fronts: to our *own* space and to the space of the forest." And in order to create that balance, both foci must be maintained simultaneously lest one overtakes the other. This is a task that can only be tackled *individually* if we are to create internal balance. We can consider and attend the needs and preferences of those around us, but we *cannot* expect "clean" support from them, free of their own personal agendas, whether conscious or not. No. This must be done on our own. And when we arrive at a place where we have become "actualized," there will be *no doubt as to who we are and what we are capable of. This* is the root and the beginning of all *Self-Trust* and *Confidence*.

We now move on to what I call *Small & Easy Steps*. I've started with the simplest steps first. Steps 1 through 5 addresses what we can do by ourselves free of the personal agendas of others; that is, free of their opinions, preferences and needs. Since our actions only involve our own independent efforts, the lack of the opinions and involvement of others will have a minimal effect on our chosen actions, choices and our ability to maintain consistency in our motivation. This will have the effect of allowing our *Self-Trust and Confidence* to build almost solely as a result of our own independent efforts. It's when we get to steps 6 and 7 that we begin to get a little more involved in dealing with the responses of others, which, in addition to childhood programming, seems to pose the primary reinforcement of what discourages us. Let's begin with the first five ways for accomplishing our simplest changes within *Small & Easy Steps*.

Small & Easy Steps

Rather than assuming the general perspective held by the public, looking at our goals as large and insurmountable endeavors requiring painfully excessive amounts of energy to overcome, there are many much simpler and easier ways to follow through on making our desired emotional individuality and stability come to fruition. Each journey can begin with ways I will call *Small & Easy Steps*, which will support and enhance the new journey. Following are a few of the small and easy step options.

Step One – USE SELF-TALK

Often times, and maybe we've already done it ourselves, we hear people talking to themselves as if someone else were speaking encouraging words about what they're doing. It may take the form of a repetitive statement or an ad lib conversation with the part of themselves that has a desire. The repetitive statement is what our contemporary metaphysical or religious communities call an *affirmation*. The ad lib conversation is not. The basic gist of the *affirmation* is that if we say it sometimes often enough we'll, first, start to believe it, and then create enough momentum through applying our energy and intentions to draw an experience that will make the thought a self-fulfilling prophesy. This may seem a little far-fetched, but it does have its merit. This is based largely on the belief that sounds and words have a vibratory power in themselves (and they do) and that they will attract "like" things to themselves, which they also do. We've all heard the saying "Birds of a feather flock together," which we've certainly seen in action. However, I'd like to make a distinction between the commonly held assumption about an *affirmation* and *Self-Talk* and how they actually play out.

An *affirmation* is usually a four or five word statement such as "I love myself" or "I am a strong and confident person." The first problem with an *affirmation* lies in the fact that we, actually, *don't* believe these things about ourselves. Usually, the original *feeling* and *thought* about ourselves that we "paired" and committed to memory early on contradicts what we want to *affirm* about ourselves. Otherwise, why would we feel the need to affirm it in the first place? ("Pairing" is explained more fully in the *Feelings, Thoughts & Emotions* section) It's important to know that what we *believe* about ourselves is what we allow ourselves to actually act on. The second difficulty is that the statement is usually too far from our perceived truth about ourselves to gain any momentum. The fact that we don't believe it makes it easy to recognize its probable nose dive. The fact that it is too far from the truth needs a little more explanation.

The statement "I am a strong and confident person" is a very broad and sweeping statement. Even when we say it, it's obvious to us that we don't actually believe it, based on the fact that we have the need to say it in the first place. However, if we were to say "I know I haven't done this in the past, but I think I might be able to handle it just this one time," we would stand a much better chance at convincing ourselves to act, simply due to the fact that it allows for the possibility of failure, but it *also* includes the potential hope for success. In saying it this way, it doesn't seem so far from our perceived truth about ourselves. Also, when we say it to ourselves in this way, the distance between what we believe about ourselves and what we want to do doesn't seem as far as it did in the *affirmation*. The statement is more specific to the situation and bites off a smaller piece of challenge. When we start any journey, don't we start off with a few simple steps? Don't we build momentum with each succeeding step? Why shouldn't changing something in ourselves work the same way as starting something new – slowly, with baby steps, and building momentum?

So our *Self-Talk* should be situation specific, *not* general and sweeping like an *affirmation*. We should address the situation gradually, a little at a time allowing for the momentum and our confidence to build slowly through our actions and resulting experience. All our experiences validate what we *feel* about ourselves and our "paired" *feeling* and *thought*, old or newly formed, determines what we will allow ourselves to act on in the future.

There is one other aspect of *Self-Talk* that needs to be recognized. It's the fact that it is *SELF* talk. There is no one else involved to produce doubt or inadequacy; no one to offer "destructive" criticism or discouragement. It's all on us. And *no one else need know* what we are challenging ourselves with. If we don't accomplish what we set out to do the first time, there is no need to contend with feeling the *shame* we might feel if others knew we "didn't make the mark." We have a clear field to make another attempt if needed.

So, use your *Self-Talk* to inch up on your goal little by little, in small steps, in little pieces. And don't tell anyone what you're doing so you don't hear flack if it doesn't, at first, turn out the way you wanted or expected. Give yourself some breathing room! This will begin to rebuild your *Self-Trust and Confidence* and slowly edge out old destructive beliefs about yourself *without* the interference of others.

Exercise #1

As with any new project, and reclaiming your *Self-Trust* truly is an important and vital project for revitalizing your self-worth; a journey begins with the first step. This first step must have a quality of tangibility for it to be recognized and acknowledged by your mind and in your world as a viable and distinguishable part of your activities in order to be considered as actually having an influence on your life. Looking back at the example of clearing a space in the forest we will now add the planting of a seedling in that space. This can be compared to military action in the establishing of a beachhead on enemy shores in order to gain a foothold in a hostile territory. Then, while your actions protect it from outside assault, you may strengthen its roots and foliage so that it may be allowed the time and nourishment to become strong enough to stand on its own amidst the external worldly chaos.

I would like you to pick some activity that you can work with physically, yet, easily and that would slip into your daily routines unnoticed by others and with no disclosure, on your part, of your participation in it with others. Set aside only one hour per week on a *specific day* clear of other activities that you regard as essential for your survival. The time of day or location is not as important as the fact that you *will* do it and not put it off in favor of other activities. It can be done three in the morning if you wish. This will be something that you have wanted to do but, owing to circumstances "beyond your control" have been unable or even unwilling to devote your time or effort into its creation. This activity will also be something that you have either not participated in before or have had minimal exposure toward experiencing it. It can be an activity like writing, archery, skating, singing, playing an instrument or something that you might physically do, build experience with and have a clear perspective of your successes and failures with it. You WILL NOT discuss or expose the fact that you're doing this activity with your family, closest friends or people that will be able to pass knowledge of your participation on to them.

This activity does not have to be large or grand in your world of activity gobbling up your time and effort while syphoning off the energy you need to survive and take care of your daily obligations. Remember, you're simply planting a seedling in the forest in the space that you've cleared. Keep it simple and discrete. We will do more with this activity later. It will represent the tangible "outing" of your confidence and projection of your new self onto the world.

Step Two – EMULATE A SUCCESSFUL CHARACTER

If we look at successful people who are either in the career we've chosen or have been successful at something we have an interest in, we can find personal traits in them that resonate with ours and allow ourselves to speculate that if they could be successful, so could we. As with *Self-Talk*, we can allow ourselves to believe that it's possible as long as we also allow for the *possibility* that it might not be. For a more complete investigation, we can read the biographies of notable people in our field in order to "stack the deck" with more specific information contributing toward the building of a believable *vision* that we may have *Self-Trust and Confidence* in pursuing for ourselves. In observing and reading about these people, their life styles and experience of success, and through building a familiarity and a feeling of similarity with them we can allow ourselves to get *closer* to *believing,* or at least allowing ourselves to *hope,* that we might have the same potential.

There are many ways in which we can connect to feeling what our successful character might feel. We can listen or watch interviews or movies they might have been in. We can read articles by them or about them. If we have enough information about them we can eat the same foods, wear the same kinds of clothing, do the same kinds of extra-curricular activities. The possibility of using our *Self-Talk* about similarities found through familiarity with them now brings our potential for success a lot closer than the first perceived distant "hero." In psychological terms, emulating the biographical path of a successful person is an alternate way of regaining more of an *internal locus of control.* And again, there is no one to discourage us. We are free to create our own experience producing the feelings of *Self-Trust and Confidence* without the interference of outsiders.

Step Three – DO THE RESEARCH

To a lesser degree, at least initially, our own curiosity into a subject may have spurred a quest for information and understanding, if only to fulfill or dispel a hunger for awareness about something that has been sparked in our interest. Whether it is a rekindled interest from a "past life" or simply an interest sparked through someone for whom we have respect, it resonated with something in us and drew our attention. These usually only surfaces if we, at the least, have had a passing attentiveness to our own *intuitive* voice. That intuitive voice is *intimately* connected to and validated by our *Self-Trust* and *Confidence.* It is often buried by childhood self-diminishing programming leaving us with only an external path determined for us by others.

When I say *Do the Research* I mean exploring more than just our field of interest. If I have an interest in learning archery, it's obvious that I will get information by going on line or purchasing magazines or catching videos or TV shows about the subject or even just buying a bow and quiver and fooling with it in my back yard or park. Getting in any field is a lot more than just the information and equipment. There is a whole Gestalt of contingent influences that can be explored and felt. For example, the ranges used for practicing alone have a "feel" about them that permeates what we perceive. There are tournaments, outings, groups that get together and destinations that color everything about the field.

We must also plan how we are going to approach our involvement. We'd research places that practice what we want to get involved with and journey to be "on site" to "feel" the environment. We, also, have to look at what is needed to participate. For example *do* we need equipment? Do we have to adjust our schedule to participate? What routines and patterns must we adjust to put ourselves "in play?" Who or what might be standing in our way? Do we have a family or other obligations that absorb the time and resources that we need to participate?

Finally, is our interest what we *really* feel inclined to do or be or is it the result of cultural or familial obligations that we might get involved with simply to avoid pressure from them or gain their approval? Remember, we have been trained to please others at our own expense. This takes a good hard look at recognizing what makes *us* happy and what our talents and leanings need for *their* expression. Most people who are active and successful in a field are often separate from family dynamics where family members have a say or influence. It is a rare occasion that a family works well together without coercive undercurrents or influences. The point here is that, again, our research is not subject to the judgment of "outsiders" unless we divulge our intentions. There is little potential for ridicule or self-diminishing.

Exercise #2

With doing the research for step three I would like you to purchase some sort of a notebook where you might document your research and the facts about the field or endeavor that you have chosen to pursue *without* the knowledge of those in your family or of your closest friends. This will serve two purposes. First, it will give you a tangible record of your efforts which will appeal to your sense of worldly logic and will supply the evidence needed for your mind to accept and acknowledge that you actually are doing this activity and that it is not to be regarded as a passing fancy. Second, this written journal, if we can call it such, will serve as a timeline and tangible measure of your progress so you may look back at the distance and knowledge that you have traversed in creating a field of endeavor that will amplify and strengthen your *Self-Trust & Confidence* in your abilities. Third, reason two will also give you the *feel* of being successful which is so necessary to sustaining any beliefs about ourselves.

Step Four - FIND A SPONSOR

One step beyond having a biographical example to read about is having a successful sponsor or advisor to "feel into" and to ask questions of directly, giving us the understanding that they are *just like us* except that they are more connected to their *Self-Trust and Confidence* than we are. A biographical book can only impart so much compared to a living person who can provide a more fully rounded and integrated example in which we might see some part of our future selves.

In addition to the possibility of a more compete model of the qualities we want to activate within ourselves, our advisor may also provide encouragement. As a note here, it is important to be cautious of the defense mechanism, *projection*, as we may attribute positive qualities in ourselves to our sponsor or model in an effort not to have to fulfill those potentials within ourselves and thereby avoid changing the inertial emotional patterns needed to accommodate them. And a big difference between this step and our previous ones is our renewed susceptibility to external influence in asking for assistance. In this step it is crucially important to have a clear *realistic* awareness of our sponsor's effect on us. A negative response from *their* personal agenda could have devastating consequences for our fledgling *Self-Trust and Confidence* development. It would probably be best to wait until we've been on our new path for a while and had some time in building our new momentum before we subjected ourselves to outside reflection. As with any new creative project, especially within reach of potential naysayers, it's better *not* to divulge our intentions until they've gained some strength and momentum. That way what we attract back from our universe is clear of influence from other co-creators (remember, birds of a feather).

Step four is the first step where we're inviting the input from others. Along with the obvious conscious input comes another dynamic which is the rarely perceived involuntary phenomenon: *empathy*. Whether it is in our consciousness or below the threshold of our awareness, empathy is *always* occurring. The challenge for us is to recognize when contact with another individual creates a change in our feelings and emotions. This can be done easily if we have prepared ourselves for recognition. I call it *taking our temperature*. The following exercise illustrates how to do this.

Exercise #4

If you are anticipating attending a business or family event where feelings and emotions may run an undesirable course, it would be best to pause, either in the parking lot or just outside the event. Sit or stand quietly and close your eyes for a few moments and let your current feelings and emotions wash over you. Pay close attention and describe to yourself, as clearly as you can, what and how your feelings and emotions are at the moment. When you've got a good handle on what you feel proceed into the event paying attention to what you begin to feel that is *different* from what you described to yourself before you entered the new environment and encountered other people. Pay attention because, at the least, you will feel a subtle shifting in how you feel. If the feeling is different from when you initially *took your temperature* before you entered, and most likely it will be, you can be assured that the new feeling is *not yours* but what you are empathizing from others in the new environment. You can also be reasonably assured that it is not your reaction to the new people in the environment because in your quiet time outside the event you were most likely aware of whom it is you would be contacting. This simple exercise helps you to separate your feelings from those you empathize.

Since our ability to empathize is involuntary we are always "ingesting" environmental feelings projected and felt by others and, more often than not, assume that they are of our own generation. Then we are faced with the impossible task of attempting to uncover why we now feel what we feel with no perceivable cause. *Taking our temperature* averts being beset with this conundrum.

In lieu of having a sponsor, we may also seek out individuals with similar interests, if not for the social component, which is a very strong draw, then simply for the information available to us merely by asking those whom we have befriended. Here is one word of caution, however. Even though we may attract those of a similar interest, we may also attract those of similar limitation. This may produce a feeling of "safety in numbers," insulating us from exerting risk by virtue of accepting a group perceived inadequacy. In other circles we would call this commiseration, which allows for a bonding that reinforces our limitations. It is imperative that our awareness must be fully in play in order that we may see through any group rationalizations leading to hurtful and limiting self-deception.

All of these steps have the power to minimize the paralyzing inaction inherent in our emotional *inertia* and bypass the harmful effects of outside judgment. At this point I need to emphasize the power behind *simple* focus. That is, *choosing* to think about things that will empower our *motivation*. I cannot stress enough the devastating effects of focusing on what is *not believed to be possible* as a cloaked encouragement toward emotional inertia by the part of us that we perceive as inadequate or inferior. It will take some time and effort to train ourselves to continually, over and over, refocus on subjects that will expand our effectiveness rather than focusing on what we have been *unable* to do in the past due to the paralyzing effects of our own toxic conditioning. Energy follows thought. The ancient Chinese said that to focus on our enemy or all the reasons we have learned why we *can't* do something, gives them power over us. Simply refocus. Remember that belief is *still* the result of our *personal experience* following a *personal* choice. Through our new *Small & Easy Steps* we will slowly forge a new set of experiences that will allow us to validate our *Self-Trust & Confidence* and build personal power in them through our renewed focus on positive and constructive endeavors *free of the limiting effects of our past conditioning willingly provided us by others!*

Step Six – USE *"I-DIALOGUE"*

Using *I-Dialogue* is a very simple thing to do, but the devil is in maintaining our awareness and keeping it active while we're moving through our daily lives. Simply put, it is taking responsibility-driven conversations that relate to people as *you, yours, they, theirs* and *them* and replacing them with *I, we, mine, ours* and *us*. At first glance this may seem to be a superficial, shallow and maybe even useless thing to do. But, don't let its simplicity fool you. Based on principles from NLP (*Neuro-Linguistic Programming*), it is a method called *reframing*. What *reframing* does is change the *context* of how perceive a subject, situation or person so we may relate to it differently, thereby changing the perspective of how we view ourselves in relation to it (them). This sounds convoluted but let me explain.

Think about the mind, the *ego* and what gives us our ability to process and store experience (covered in more depth in the Layman's Perspective section). The mind's main method of sorting and classifying the subject is by separating what it encounters into individual parts so it can compare and contrast them. Then it can create and commit to memory decisions about them based on its judgments and assessments so we can have a response prepared for handling the subject or situation in the future. Its main tool for doing this is its ability to sort and separate. Our *ego* is simply a structure created by the mind. It also uses sorting and separating to classify its experience so it can use the information to identify itself. Its main tool for protecting and identifying itself is its set of *defense mechanisms*. Its primary mechanism is *projection* - attributing to others what it is that we find difficult in acknowledging or accepting about ourselves. To create that distance or separation when dealing with people we use words like *you, yours, they, theirs* and *them*. Once we have separated ourselves from others, all that remains is the simple task of depositing our perceived unwanted qualities on *them*. This is the essence of *projection*. In our minds, the responsibility for dealing with those qualities now lies with *them*. So, through using words of separation - *you, yours, they, theirs* and *them* - we have, effectively, distanced ourselves from and absolved ourselves of being responsible for qualities that we privately believe we have that are undesirable. Now, back to *I-Dialogue*.

If we substitute *I, we, mine, ours* and *us* in situations where responsibility is the focus and where we feel inclined to use the words *you, yours, they, theirs* and *them*, we will effectively short circuit our ability to *project* our undesirable qualities onto others through distancing ourselves from them. Why would we want to do that, you might ask? First, by addressing others in the first person we eliminate our ability to distance ourselves from them. Second, if there is no distancing or separation, we are unable to use *projection* to divest ourselves of the qualities we *believe* that we possess, wish to deny, and prefer not to deal with. That is, we are unable to attribute to others what we prefer not to accept about ourselves. And third, by doing this these qualities and issues now become unavoidable and look us squarely in the face. We now can see them clearly for what they are - ours and needing to be acknowledged, accepted and handled. There is no escaping ourselves if we want to excel through feeling *Self-Trust* and *Confidence*. How does doing this help?

There is another deeper dimension activated by doing this, and is our reason for doing it this way. It puts us in a position of having to be *accountable*. To accept and change something about ourselves we must first *own it*. This shift helps us to do just that, in allowing us to become aware of its existence within us and be *accountable* for "it" and the consequences it produces. Using *projection* enables us to disown it and place it instead with the person who is responsible for making us expose and face it. Relating to others through changing the pronoun reduces or even eliminates our potential for distancing ourselves from them and what we must deal with. We have, essentially, *reframed* the situation by changing the *context* moving from perceiving our undesirable quality as being *outside* ourselves to being *inside* ourselves, or within *our* domain and under *our* control.

In doing this something else occurs. With external *locus of control* we believe that the world controls our fate. With internal *locus of control* we believe it is within *our* control. So, in light of what we've done with *I-Dialogue*, to *own* what we *didn't* want to believe or accept about ourselves is now *within our power to change it*.

Accountability

We all have at least a minimal number of differences in the way we see or feel being *accountable*. For our purposes here, I will say that for us to be *accountable* only requires that we simply acknowledge that we made and acted on a personal choice(s) based on *our own* personal assessments and values. It in no way implies that we must adjust it, fix it, ease someone else's distress about it, or somehow change the circumstances surrounding it. Unfortunately, this appears to be the perspective that most Westerners seem to feel naturally follows an admission of *accountability*: an assumed progression into being "responsible" for its effects and an obligation to adjust, fix, change, or ease someone else's objection to our deed if it is uncomfortable or distressing to them. This works in conjunction with the social expectation that if we do, act, or be what we desire without first considering how it will affect others, we will be considered and labeled *selfish*. (Read the post *The Taboo Against Being & Taking What We Desire* on *www.JohnMaerz.com/EmotionalTroubleshooter*.)

In our culture, the words *blame, responsibility* and *accountability* have all somehow taken on the same meaning. From this perspective, its contemporary meaning tends to lend itself very nicely to the dynamic of *projection*; pushing it away from us and applying its social label and assumed obligation onto someone else. In other words, in *blaming* others, or in this case, making others *accountable* for our deeds, we essentially absolve ourselves from having to accept the social label of "bad" or *selfish* and assign it and the requirement of having to "pay restitution," whether monetarily, emotionally, or socially, to someone else. With everyone assuming different levels of responsibility in different circumstances we can see how overwhelmingly confusing our individual assignations and expectations can become.

I-Dialogue helps us to bring our stored and harmful childhood *self-worth* triggers to the surface by accepting our complicity in the *current* experience and keeping it conscious while we pair it again, through *reframing* the experience, with new *thoughts* (self-assessments) and *feelings* different from the dysfunctional ones that we previously learned, attributed and submerged. This is how it works. Once we have acknowledged our actions as the result of our own decisions, they remain, with clarity, within our awareness, enabling us to assess them and compare them to our *current* perception of ourselves based on our *new* perceptions, judgments and feelings about the *current* experience. The ambiguity of our past childhood programming about our *self-worth* is now out in the open and easily compared with our *current* circumstances and is allowed a fresh observation in a new perspective. This, effectively, allows us to pair new *thoughts* and assessments with the triggered memory of the past experience replacing the old previously repressed and damaging judgments about our *self-worth* we accepted as a child.

I-Dialogue puts the *accountability* for our actions squarely on our shoulders by preventing our ability to distance ourselves from them. However, we still, unfortunately, have to deal with the assumption of others that we are obligated to do something about them. Although this perspective is often negotiable with others depending on what they expect to gain from it, we must be exceedingly cautious not to accept or agree to any obligation that might lead to accepting a judgment or assessment of *our* character based on *their* values and experiences. They have a right to feel about us as they wish but should not be allowed to determine our *self-worth*. Nevertheless, there will still remain those who are unmovable in their opinion of how we should behave or act in spite of, or even in lieu of, their experience with us. This is just a fact of life. *We all choose what to believe and expect based on our prior individual experience.* But, at least in applying *I-Dialogue* we can become aware of the new circumstances that have presented themselves relative to what we are about to decide about ourselves so we can revisit similar prior experiences and reassess ourselves in light of what we may have learned since having them. The most important point to take away from *I-Dialogue* and *accountability* is that they enable us to reduce or eliminate the influence of others on how we judge ourselves. This becomes a major factor in changing our acclimation to and viewing of life and its circumstances from an external *locus of control* to an internal *locus of control*, the most important component in enabling us to use our *Self-Trust and Confidence* over socially and externally applied judgments about our *self-worth*.

There is still one aspect of *I-Dialogue* that I would like to cover before we move on. Changing the pronouns might sometimes sound rather strange to us when we apply this process to *all* the situations involving them. Our target for using *I-Dialogue* is to intercept only those situations that involve our *accountability* and issues of responsibility. But not all situations involving its use do so. Let me explain.

It would make sense that in sharing a task to be completed in a work environment, that if there was an issue to work out, for us to ask what *we* are going to do about it rather than asking our coworker what *you* are going to do about it. Usually, asking someone what are *you* going to do about something, more often than not, puts them on the defensive by making them feel vulnerable to potential criticism. In any shared work environment there are almost always tasks involving needed complicity. The *we* helps us to stay focused on the issues and not be distracted by involving ourselves in the need to highlight placing blame or responsibility. Making it a cooperative effort enables flexibility in *accountability*, for *both* workers, while relieving potential threats of exposure or accusations of inadequacy.

In another situation where there is work that is supposed to be completed by those in a common environment and it isn't, asking what *we* are going to do about it distributes the responsibility and eliminates the potential for blame by offering cooperation. This drops defenses and makes the work not only easier but perceivable as a combined responsibility. Then, even if either you or your coworker have concerns about your own adequacy or competency, making it a cooperative effort eliminates the potential of reinforcing any perceived inadequacies with the threat of exposure leading to blaming.

In the two above examples, friendship may serve as a setting for the same kinds of situations but, due to the fact that friendship is involved, both parties often find it easier to forgive any inequalities or personal shortcomings of the other by virtue of the nurturing quality of the friendship.

Extracting Ourselves from Manipulative Influence

Now, here's the biggest challenge as we change the focus from them to you. In a home or family environment competition for dominance or authority that lends itself to cloaking the exposure of believed inadequacy may be a lot more intense and overt than experienced in the work environment. Dysfunctional family structures are a lot more likely to be strongly and deeply ingrained, keeping any patterns of *projection* well in place in order to keep responsibility, *accountability* and inadequacy firmly *projected* on a specific member of a family. Additionally, there is a loyalty and discretion expected of that family member to remain silent about relevant issues with those outside the family. This can be experienced subtlety or in a very blatant form. We realize this is true in more extreme but inferred circumstances when we hear things like, "Oh, Uncle Harry has always been lazy" or "Little Jimmy has never been able to stay straight with the law." The *projected* dysfunctions maintain the focus on one member of the family as being the root or cause of why the family group has been unable to "make the grade" or excel in normal experiences expected of an average family. This keeps the focus of inadequacy, incompetency or fear of failing off the other members of the family who will, now, never have to put forth any effort to excel. They have an excuse not to perform. They may then proceed through life blameless for not taking the risk to participate in needed life experiences.

Changing our use of the pronouns in the more serious scenarios with those who have assigned us permanent *accountability* for a defect will meet with tremendous resistance if not overt antagonism, especially since we're including the assigners a place within the scope of responsibility. Dysfunctional family structures remain consistent only by continually reassigning blame for their difficulties to specific family members with an obvious "defect" in order to keep the dysfunction alive and in place. When threatened with accountability for failed *family* performance, whether through changed pronouns or something a little more obtuse, they will resort emotional blackmail through threatening the "defective" member with the cessation of continuing their family support in some fashion. This may show itself as the withdrawal of love or expressing the "inability" to do something for us that was promised. When we forgo what was promised to us or inferred, tacitly or openly we remove the power they hold over us. This is the first step in subtly disconnecting their controlling influence. In doing this we slowly remove ourselves from allowing them to use us as a scapegoat in using us to cover their own perceived inadequacies.

There are many families that have a relatively normal rapport but, more often than not, we find these kinds of control scenarios prevalent even in the most respected of families. Think of the publicity a famous person or family gains when this kind of blame assignment comes to public knowledge via a scandal. The pattern is not different in smaller social contexts, just a little less widespread. Our *egos* are *extremely* resourceful when defending themselves. In play, also, is the axiom that *no one does anything for just one reason*. All *motivations* come with more than one reason for acting and with options and variations. We are multilevel creatures slipping from level to level depending on where the social and material benefits are best. *Accountability* short circuits a lot of the ambiguities and our ability to "change sides" in order to save face. Changing pronouns is a small step in making clarity and *accountability* a reality.

Changing pronouns makes it painfully obvious to those *projecting* blame that there is a growing resistance to allowing them to maintain the illusion of being competent and in charge, i.e. dictating our behavior. It often elicits vehement objections. But that vehemence occurs only temporarily and remains in the moment. What becomes more tragic is the temperament it produces in a child subject to these kinds of manipulation. The younger the child, the more harmful and ingrained the feeling of inadequacy and incompetence grows. *Self-Trust and Confidence* become severely diminished if not extinguished. As we grow beyond a child into an adult, we are most likely to continue to believe that we are in some way inadequate by becoming a self-fulfilling prophesy through attracting relationships that refill the role of the abuser that we grew up with. *Shame* and feelings of inadequacy then become perpetuated. This totally extinguishes *motivation*.

It's important to realize that in changing pronouns outside of our family we are not only making it more comfortable for many of those we connect with to feel the absence of any threat of criticism or for the exposure of any perceived inadequacies, but we are also setting the foundation for our own sense of responsibility by keeping our *accountability* right up front and allowing no ambiguity of circumstance while also keeping us away from the temptation to blame. It's important too, to realize that any changes that we make in ourselves are more easily done and maintained with people far from the center of our usual participation with others. Friends may be a little more challenging due to our frequency of contact and history but perhaps a bit more tolerant and understanding based on the depth of friendship. Family members are the most upset and often can become the most ornery and downright abusive in reacting to our new presentation of ourselves and our attempted adjustments to our relationships with them. Is it any wonder that the old adage "a prophet is not a prophet in their own home town" is so widely known and understood?

A Word of Caution When Using *I-Dialogue*

Moving back to changing our pronouns, we can see how some of us may react mildly to the changes and others may be totally self-consumed by their feelings and the fear of being exposed, whether a belief about their inadequacy is imagined or justified. What we must look at is *when* to use *I-Dialogue*. We have to be the judge of when to shift *accountability*. *Always* changing the pronouns may end up sounding rather ludicrous in some cases and draw some really strange looks from the people we do it with. So we must be mindful in restricting our own use to situations that *only* involve responsibility and *accountability*. This may sometimes be difficult to assess and there is always present a "slippery slope" with the temptation for us to use it in assigning responsibility to others for things we should be addressing ourselves. The biggest hazard is that this process can work both for us and against us. In this light it can become a double standard by using the practice as a *projection*. So a word of caution, make certain that you are being honest with yourself and not just shifting blame.

Working with *I-Dialogue* and using the first five *Small & Easy Steps* is a very strong and effective beginning. But at some point we will return to the scrutiny and observation by others of who we are and what we do. When we do we will have to have a solid grounding in who we are, what we want and how we have rebuilt our *Self-Trust* and *Confidence.* This will be no easy task as our *ego* will go a long way to defend itself even if it kills our own ability for action in doing so. To this end we must develop a strategy to handle personal interchanges that will attempt to push us back into roles that support others' impressions, visions and expectations of us. Just because we have made the internal changes needed does not mean that we will not have to defend our new position with others. The up side is that this will be easy to do with strangers. The down side is that it will be very difficult to do with family and those with which we have had a history of dependency and close emotional rapports. The temptation to continue to want a sense of belonging with and approval of others will seem overwhelming in the face of threatened excommunication by those who fear exposure by us of their sometimes not so subtle manipulations of our behavior to maintain the suppression of their own perceived feelings of inadequacy. It's not that these are "bad" people. We all have at least some of these *feelings* and almost all of us have reacted instinctually to keep these feelings covered. Most of us have had the experiences and reinforcement that produced these *feelings* so long ago that they are deeply submerged and the *ego* has strategized defensive actions that have become almost entirely unconscious and instinctual. We might say that "some of us can't help ourselves," which might be a very pessimistic outlook on our potential, but fits the current perspective fueled by our past experiences until we can get a handle on intercepting and reprogramming our tendency to act without awareness. But changing others is not our responsibility. Falling into being accountable for that is another one of the strategized traps…even if it is unconscious. No, our task is to untangle ourselves from the emotional collusion that has held us captive for so long. We will have to devise a way of recognizing when the *accountability* is actually ours and when it is being used by others as a ploy to re-establish our support for their cover. With others, especially with family members and those close to us with whom we have a history, we can clarify our position ahead of time by asking ourselves a series of questions. These will expose our assumed and assigned obligations and responsibilities for maintaining dysfunctionality. In many cases this will result in an unspoken power play that will almost certainly result in some form of excommunication for us when we act from the perspective that we have come to understand through our questioning. Our questions are intended to clarify what we believe we are expected to be responsible and *accountable* for, and who is doing the expecting - us or them.

Rather than following the usual line of questioning that most self-help books utilize which is "What do I really want?" I will pursue a line of questioning which will focus on where our power and permissiveness comes from relative to the people we feel are important in our lives. I've chosen to do it this way because what usually happens when we follow the "What do I really want?" path is that it yields answers that address and appease the authority figures we were raised by. That is, the things we *say* and *think* that we want are usually geared, even if unconsciously, toward satisfying the rules and requirements that we were indoctrinated with when we were children. These usually work with and include adhering to the self-diminishing judgments and characteristics that put us into our current dysfunctional relationship problems in the first place. What's unfortunate is that our feelings, which often have been buried early on, disagree with what our social doctrines tell us we *should* want. What we usually *say* and *think* we want are to be productive, be a good father or mother, contribute to society and a whole host of things that address the needs of the world *outside* of our inner sphere. What we *really* want is love, affection, approval, to be listened to, to be encouraged, to simply have *our* needs considered and maybe even answered by others, and all the things we say we want to be able to do and give to others…like we've been trained to "want."

If I can put this in another way, my focus is to reduce our tendency toward supporting an exterior *locus of control* and toward building and then reinforcing *more* of an internal *locus of control. Note, I said more of, not instead of* – that extreme would be just as badly out of balance. In short, it's to help us see who we've put in charge of directing our lives and why. This line of questioning is also geared toward preventing us from regurgitating our trained responses that maintain our current dysfunctional status quo which has *been continually and repeatedly reinforced over our personal needs and desires* by the world through keeping us preoccupied with being our brother's keeper.

So, now that I have given you the focus of the questions and why I've chosen that focus; let's move on to working with the questions themselves. Please find a quiet space and a quiet time so you may allow yourself enough space and privacy to deal with the questions honestly. Make sure you don't sabotage your efforts by setting yourself up in a scenario to do this where you will be assaulted by your family, the telephone, business needs or bodily functions. You must be in a space that is free of the imposing needs of others. Let's proceed.

I think it's obvious that the people who are on our minds the most are the people who have the most influence over us. Those of us who might be little older may no longer have our parents with us, however it is almost a certainty that some time after their loss we will have slipped someone else into their position to continue the rapport and continuity of their support, or not, that we had when they *were* in our lives. After all, we are creatures of habit and don't respond to change well. We almost always recreate our situations over and over to give our lives consistency and familiarity to assure our feelings of comfort and security.

Please answer these list #1 questions as thoughtfully and honestly as you can even if you feel as if your answers may seem hurtful to you or those you name. It may also be possible that there may be more than one person to which the qualification is applicable. Do your best to choose the one who *best* fits the question. This will make things a little easier for you when you determine how to handle them and others like them in the future. If you split the qualification between different individuals it may water down, or defocus, or scatter your needed future intent. Also, please answer these six questions *before* you read on. If you don't, your answers will be qualified, or tainted through being warned how they will apply to you, and you'll miss out on some very valuable self-insights.

List #1 - PEOPLE

1. The most important person in my life is____________.

2. The most unimportant person in my life is__________.

3. The person I love the most is______________________________.

4. The person I dislike or hate the most is______________.

5. The person I envy the most is______________________.

6. The person I fear the most is______________________.

Most of us will answer the first question, the most *important*, with a person that we think may have the most *positive* influence on how we are living our current story. For those of us who are married or have a long term relationship, the person named will most often be the same. We may name our spouse or partner because they actually *are* the most important or we may answer because we think that they *should* be. Which one is the most important to us is not as important as the fact that we picked them as such. These people serve as the baseline for how we believe we want to or should be living our lives. They represent our face toward the world. They represent what it is that we openly acknowledge about ourselves *to* ourselves.

Most of us will answer the second question, the most *unimportant*, first with difficulty, since we'd be questioning ourselves relative to whom we might be inattentive to or have little or no acknowledgement of their influence over our lives, but also with puzzlement as to why they would even be included in an assessment of *our* world. These people represent our *unconscious shadow*. They represent the qualities in ourselves that we have little or no knowledge of or have buried far from the surface because they represent a serious threat to how we see ourselves. But we might say, "But they're unimportant. How can they have an influence over me?" And the answer would be, "Because you picked *them* over all the other people who have little or no importance for you. It is them that you picked. Why them?" That alone says that they have significance.

Most of us will answer the third question, who we *love* the most, as the person having the qualities we most admire and love about *ourselves*. But you may say, "But I love them because *they* have those qualities." And you'd be right. But since like attracts like or "birds of a feather flock together," is a basic rule of the natural universe, *you* also have the qualities that you are assigning to the person you most love. They may not be necessarily being expressed by you at the moment but to recognize a quality in someone you must first possess it within yourself or at least have had firsthand experience with it. Our most cherished relationships reflect our inner qualities the best regardless of whether we are expressing them or not.

At this point, after you've read and understood how question three relates to you, you're probably saying to yourself, "I know what's coming with question four." And you'd be right. The qualities the person you most hate or dislike has are those qualities within yourself that you most hate or dislike and would like to do all you can to distance yourself from. These qualities represent your *conscious shadow*. Think about the people you criticize the most harshly and you will see the things within you that are either unresolved or have the most detrimental effect on the image you'd like to *project* toward the *outside* world. The more strongly you deny or *project* those qualities on others the more deeply you feel that they are a part of you.

Question five is interesting: Who you *envy* the most? Who you envy does not represent who you are actually jealous of but who has the qualities that you admire about yourself that you feel you have been unable or unwilling to express or bring out of yourself. Usually, the circumstances that surround the quality you envy, feel threatening or unachievable are so because of how you must change or what you must deal with within yourself in order to express them. For example, to be envious of someone who is courageous, means that first, that you do possess the quality, otherwise you wouldn't have recognized it and, second, that you would have to somehow change yourself and move outside your comfort zone in order to express it. That means that your relationship with others would have to go through a change also. They might come to expect this of you. Then what would you do if you couldn't make the grade again? This is the unknown horizon. This is the reason that fear of success is more intense than the fear of failure. Everyone is familiar with failure, and commiseration with others is an easy option. But fear of success challenges our *Self-Trust* and *Confidence*. For many of us, that is unknown territory and there is no one there to commiserate with. We're all alone. Often, there is more security in the devil we do know than the devil in what we don't. So, it's just easier to apply the enviable quality to someone else rather than risk our security in what we might not be able to keep up with. And yes. This *is projection*, not over what we don't want, but what we feel we can't be, do or continue. We're defending for the failure of being a possible success. Twisted, isn't it? But our *ego* is extremely resourceful and devious in how it defends itself and stays within its perceivable working envelope.

Question six, who we *fear*, is similar to question five in a lot of ways in that it follows a similar dynamic, even to the point that we might envy the power another person has over us. And yes, we do have the same quality within us to make others fearful of us. However, the main focus we need to attend to here is our fear of exposure by the person we're afraid of. What do we fear? We fear the exposure of our lack of abilities and adequacy. We may also fear being harmed by another person. But that in itself is a feared inadequacy; a fear of not being able to defend ourselves whether physically or emotionally. We would most certainly not want our perceived inadequacies to become common knowledge to others. So, the person we fear somehow has the power to expose our inadequacies - either to ourselves or to others. If to others, this also gives them the potential for blackmailing us, which is exposing us to others if we act in a way that they consider undesirable for *them*. We can be easily used and abused through what we're fearful of.

An interesting side to being fearful of someone is that we may also have the power to make others fearful of *us* exposing *them*. Knowing this about ourselves, we may be tempted to do so in order to preserve our image in the face of what someone knows about us that we wish not to become common knowledge. Being fearful can be a double edged sword. We fear exposure of *our own* inadequacy by the person who wields power over us, and we can fear our own susceptibility *to being tempted* to do so to others and the consequences and self-loathing for the using of it.

Why Did We Give Them the Power?

So, now we have clarity about whom we've chosen to fill the roles in life that exemplify how we will face it. It's time to understand what those choices mean regarding how we are able to navigate the landscape we've constructed for ourselves and why we have chosen that path. I say landscape we've constructed because our personal relationships are always a reflection of what we've decided about ourselves. As a child being born and emerging into a polarized world we can only come to know ourselves through the reflection and/or responses of others to the urges and actions we experiment with in order to find or create the signposts that will define and guide us through the rest of our journey. We have only our own experience and those reflections to assess our position in the world and to become acquainted with our limits even though they are still the result of our own processing. Moving past our childhood constructed limits can only occur when we are either pushed beyond them through circumstance or we observe someone else navigating past where we have been. Let's take a look at the enveloped boundaries and assessments that we have put into place and why we chose them.

There will be many reasons that we chose someone as being the most important to us. Remember, along the same line of thinking, we *never* have only one motivation for doing anything. We are multidimensional creatures and act and react on every level, whether to support, activate or repress. Our interchange with another person also occurs on many levels. We just might not be conscious of it. Yet, it occurs nonetheless.

Obviously, what we chose as important equates to influence: that which we can exert and that which catalyzes us. Every conscious inter-personal interchange we execute will almost always have, at the least, one conscious intent. As we process what we want, more variations in what we want and how it might go appear to us. Motivations we have below our threshold of awareness may produce urges and leanings that feel non-descript. We end up saying to ourselves, "I don't know where this is coming from but I feel I should…" Often, what is expressed below our threshold of consciousness may have a purpose, also, but not something that we might be aware of at the time of expression. In this we find that our hindsight eventually informs us of what we might not have known consciously at the time but that still had play in how we made our decisions. This "below the threshold" dynamic is *always* in play when we focus on the most important person in our lives. As an analogy, what's below the water level of an iceberg may not be visible to us but its weight and position always exert an influence. Whether we eventually realize it or not depends on how much personal digging we do into our own psyche and how much and how often we might, instead, push it further below the water level.

I've separated out the people in the six questions to give us an idea of how many perspectives with which we might approach our relationships. I'm sure there are many more but these are the basic "categories" we *consciously* use to determine how and if we are going to relate with someone. If I followed each category separately and delineated how to deal with each one, we'd all be very happy thinking we have a pattern to commit to memory and an application for all the future issues that might arrive within our life sphere and path that might be similar. But we'd only be fooling ourselves. Everyone we meet and interrelate with has combinations of all of the categories and no set method is going to account or compensate for all the possible variations we will have to contend with. Every situation and interchange will be different, as are its participants…and they invariably morph depending on our followed responses. Then our plan will require a change in the rules we've chosen to govern our future behavior with them. So rather than setting up external rules that we might feel secure in proceeding with, I'd rather ask another set of questions geared to what it is we feel we might be gaining, losing, avoiding, uncovering, etc. *in the moment* with each person we are involved with in our sphere of influence. The questioning is also intended to allow us to come to an understanding of why we keep them in our space despite the fact that they may seem dangerous to maintaining or establishing our *Self-Trust* and *Confidence*.

So, why did we give them power in our sphere? Because they offer what it is that we feel we might need for the continuity of our personal beliefs, as enhancing or diminishing as they may be, which in turn solidifies the stability, or in some cases just the continuity, of our *ego*. Sometimes, even an erratic personality serves as an effective *defense mechanism*. After all, it's harder to hit a moving target!

What Do They Expect From Us?

So, now that we've blown our first coagulating structure that we could have used to sort and deal with emotional entanglements, what's left for us to regroup with? What we find about the people we've included and involved in our life path is almost always about what we *feel* when we deal with them. This invariably translates to what *we* expect of them and ourselves through interactions. What we expect is solely dependent upon the experiences we've had, with them or those before, in which we have assessed ourselves and those who might be similar to those we are dealing with so that we might be prepared for future encounters with them. What *they* expect of us can actually be, and most often is, a mystery to us. Most of us rarely *ask* what someone wants of us and we usually just *assume* what that is, based on our prior feelings and interaction with them. So, if we ask questions about what we feel, what we expect and what we anticipate doing, or not, and what we anticipate *them* doing or not, we can have a fairly good idea of what our prior experiences have produced in our belief systems that restrict or accelerate our behaviors, thereby, affecting our *motivations*.

The type of questioning we'll use is what I call the *Emotional Trail*. It will show the "pairing" (explained in depth in the *Feelings, Thoughts & Emotions* section) that we've made between our feelings and the thoughts used to create the emotional trigger that presages how we will act with or react to them. How we choose to act or react, or not, spells out the dynamic that our behavior will follow with individuals and those for whom we feel similarity.

There are a few things to know before we proceed. Please note that I've included *feelings* and *emotions* as a response for some of the blanks. Using only *feeling* characterizes only a vague or undefined response, even as intense as it might be. Emotions, because of the mental qualification that we attach to a feeling when we create an emotion, paints a much more exacting picture of what is being felt. Please also note that the last response to the questions only requires one of the seven *Elementary Feelings* of *surprise, fear, disgust, anger, happiness, sadness or apathy.* For a better understanding about *Elementary Feelings* and how they are related to and different from emotions, please read *Feelings, Thoughts & Emotions* in the *Layman's Perspective* section.

I have also purposely *not* included the word "love." For obvious reasons, the meaning of love is totally nebulous and subjective and requires more detail to understand, fully, the depth that may be intended. There are in the world as many forms of "love" that we can comprehend as there are people in the world. Additionally, words like love, OK, and fine, used relative to what we're *feeling,* tend to be catch-all words when we are unable to give a more exacting response, and should be avoided. If you must use them, do so, but be advised that these words will tend to water down the focus needed to define what it is we may be dealing with.

I have also included a list of feelings, emotions, actions and judgments in Appendix I to compensate for any "selective amnesia" we may encounter when we attempt to best describe our feelings, emotions, actions and judgments. I've also included a copy of the list of "PEOPLE" and the "EMOTIONAL TRAIL" in the appendix so you may copy them and add people if you wish or share the work with another. Remember, our *ego* is extremely clever and can also "blank the mind" if it feels threatened by where a line of thinking may be going.

Please follow through and answer the questions honestly and to the best of your ability. You've already done list #1, PEOPLE now do list #2, the EMOTIONAL TRAIL, *for each person* on your PEOPLE list completed earlier. And, again, please don't look ahead, so your approach and perspective will be fresh and untarnished by any prior knowledge.

EMOTIONAL TRAIL

1. With this person ________________ I feel the most (For E)
    ____

2. When I think about them I am (F or E) ________________ .

3. Feeling (F or E) ____________ about them makes me want to
    (A) ________________ .

4. When I imagine myself doing this I feel (F or E) ____________ .

5. When I feel (F or E)________________ I know that I am being
    (J)________________

6. Being (J)____________ I feel (F or E)____________ and I want
    to (A)____________

7. This only makes me feel ________________________________
    (Elementary Feeling ONLY)

8. Why do you think this makes you feel as you do in question #7
    ____

Chart Key: F = Feeling, E = Emotion, A = Action, J = Judgment

Now that you've filled in the blanks *for each* of your six chosen people it's time to see what you can do with them. Hopefully, you have a whole group of people whom you've assessed. Now, let's explain the process and what it can do for you.

The most important part of the Emotional Trail is question #7 as it gives you a "pairing" of each person with an elementary feeling. And each of the elementary feelings rests on a scale which extends from feeling comfortable and in control to feeling uncomfortable and out of control. Let me dive into the scale first so when we add the people you've selected it will give more insight as to the influence on how we process and establish our approach to the world and the people in it.

When I speak of feeling in control, it brings back the concept of *locus of control*. To refresh our memory, internal *locus of control* is when we feel as if *we* are in control of our life circumstances and external *locus of control* is when we feel that our life circumstances are controlled from *outside* our influence. The *Elementary Feelings* each embody qualities of both in different ratios or balance point between either extreme. On the internal side of "feeling in control" we have *happiness*. On the external side where others have control we have *fear*. The others range between the two extremes at varied points. Here is a perspective on how I see each and in what order, as follows:

Happiness – For most people happiness is a feeling of being free to be able to be and do what we want with little or no interference from the outside world. And if there is any interference, it is something that is so unimportant or irrelevant that we barely perceive it. It is the closest to our feeling of having a completely internal *locus of control*.

Surprise – It is very similar to happiness on the scale but with an element of outside play or influence making us feel that we're not quite as free or in control as we might have thought or liked. Usually, its occurrence is not of our own doing. However, it usually has a minimal dampening effect on our feeling in control.

Sadness – In *sadness* it is acknowledged that there are some circumstances in the world which are beyond our control. We *do* mind them being so but do not need to resist or challenge the experience knowing that we cannot change it. We also do not feel trapped in the experience and we know that we have other options to feel free and mobile if we choose not to react to its occurrence.

Disgust – *Disgust* is similar to *sadness* but with more of an active component. The repulsion of *disgust* resonates with the *shadow* part of us that we refuse or deny and consequently *project* on others. The rise of *disgust* triggered within us is testimony to our awareness of feeling less in control of our environment and circumstances than with *sadness* but with enough of an internal *locus of control.* to still push away our *shadow* and refocus on other options that present more of an opportunity for self-determination. Unfortunately, the ratio between internal and external *locus of control* in this case leans a little more toward the external than the internal.

Anger – *Anger* holds much of the same impetus as disgust, does but there is more of an urge to pursue the object of our *anger* with the intention of either eliminating the cause or changing the perspective of the person who, besides us, creates the tension. *Anger* is the expression of feeling our energy or direction of flow blocked, and countering the blockage with our own resistance. This resistance gains its power from our perceived immobility and failure to refocus on an easier path by virtue of our belief or assumption that external circumstances have more power and influence over our chosen path or direction than we do.

There are varying degrees of anger that we can feel, which depend on how free or blocked we may feel. The more blocked we feel, the more intense the *anger*. The *anger* itself is powered by the hope or belief that an impasse *can* be moved beyond, with either the right intensity or the right external manipulation.

Fear – *Fear* is a lot like *anger* except that its intensity is consequently turned inward as a result of the belief or assumption that the external environment is totally in control and that we have no option or ability to refocus other than to simply withdraw from, avoid or escape the situational consequences. It is the feeling that lives the furthest into the external *locus of control* perspective.

The feeling of *fear* is often tightly paired and interwoven with depression in that its most common effect is immobility, either out of fear of losing the self (physical, emotional or egotistically) or of losing or having lost an important person in our lives. Again, this is the feeling of being totally out of control. This is a feeling of helplessness which is the primary contributor to the manifestation of fear and depression and the most dominant factor in perceiving that our life operates from an external *locus of control*.

Apathy – This is the last feeling I would like to cover, which is *not* included in Ekman's pantheon of *Elementary Feelings*. I hesitate in assigning it a position in the range between internal and external *locus of control* because its flexibility allows the dynamic to be activated anywhere along the internal/external continuum depending on our resiliency and fortitude in processing the other six feelings. Let me explain.

When we think of *apathy* most of us perceive someone who doesn't care or appears to have no feelings about a situation. To this day we idolize characters like Dirty Harry who *appear* to be immune to circumstances that would have ordinarily triggered *fear, anger* or any other feelings or emotions in us, the average person. But we know that this type of *projected* persona is simply a ruse. We know that they are actually experiencing the feeling, but being "brave" or "tough" and covering the evidence of it. We even admire the ability to do so. This is the deadpan essence of a "poker face." But what about people who, honestly, no longer show the feeling, even involuntarily, through *micro-expressions*, as discussed in *Feelings, Thoughts & Emotions*? What about the people who have become so over-stimulated that they've shut down out of self-preservation? What about those who have arrived at burnout and nothing gets to them anymore; they've become totally desensitized?

The dynamic that occurs with a person who has received a traumatic physical injury can also happen as a result of an emotional trauma; we go into shock. The body shuts down. Our awareness of pain is turned off. It is my belief than anyone who has had a trauma eliciting the intensity of one of the *Elementary Feelings* beyond their personal limit or tolerance can also shut down to the point where they couldn't even be perceived in *micro-expressions*. For example, there have been people in combat situations that have elicited an extreme intensity of *fear*, yet the soldier performs a heroic action that a normal person feeling the *fear* would have been immobilized by. And then, when the soldier is asked of his deed, he *doesn't remember what he was feeling* at the time and says he could only focus on what needed to be done. Was this a ruse? I think not, in most cases. It is my belief that we could also blank out or emit an expression of *apathy*, or no *apparent* feeling, if over-stimulated, depending on whether our emotional threshold for dealing with the situation has been surpassed by external circumstances. People who are extremely depressed, autistic or even catatonic also fall into this dynamic. Essentially, we, they, withdraw from perceiving the effects of experiencing the hyper-stimulation of a feeling in order to keep it from causing irreparable damage to our current sense of who we are. Perhaps there truly are some people who commit crimes who are not aware of what they are participating in or perceiving. Our ability or tendency to "tune in" or "space out" has a vast range relative to our thresholds and tolerances for dealing with intense experiences, and each person can fall onto that scale on different points.

So, is it possible to be involuntarily *apathetic?* Sure. Remember, all *feelings* occur *involuntarily* and are not consciously changed until they are "paired" with a thought through an experience and become an emotion. Would *apathy* show in their *micro-expressions*? Most likely not, since *apathy* is the *absence* of feeling. So I think Dr. Ekman should have included *apathy* in his pantheon of *Elementary Feelings because it doesn't register* through *micro-expressions* yet it is a viable place for us to end up in dealing with our feelings. Even in music, the spaces between the notes are just as important as the notes themselves. The spaces between are invisible partners.

The Elementary Feeling Scale

An important note to understand and remember when "pairing" our *Elementary Feelings* with any one person is that those feelings can change in an instant if the circumstance involving them also changes. Also, we are not one-dimensional when it comes to our feelings. We do not experience only one feeling per person, but a combination of feelings in any given circumstance. *What we most want to focus on is how we feel **overall** when we deal with an individual.* This will give us a baseline for our attitude and rapport in dealing with them. Along the lines of giving us a baseline, we'll want to be able to *feel* some kind of sense of where the feeling actually is on the "feeling in control" scale. At the risk of being scientific or too technical I'd like to assign numbers of intensity to each *Elementary Feeling* so we have a *feel* of where we are on the scale within our perceived *locus of control*. Let's assign (+3) to **Happiness**, (+2) to **Surprise**, (+1) to **Sadness**, (0) to **Apathy**, (-1) to **Disgust**, (-2) to **Anger** and (-3) to **Fear**. What this does is tell us that when we feel *happiness*, or +3, we are feeling the *most* in control of our lives that we can be and that when we feel *fear*, or -3, we are feeling the *least* in control of our lives. With this in mind let's move on to our pairing of important people with our *Elementary Feelings* and what this means for us in how we approach life and whom we include in it.

We first started discovering who is in control with the most important person on our PEOPLE list #1. Next, we moved through our EMOTIONALTRAIL list #2 with them and were asked for our feelings, emotions, actions and judgments. On line #7 we were asked for an *Elementary Feeling* only; one of the seven. That *Elementary Feeling* corresponds to how we feel with that person the majority of our time with them. So if, for example, we feel *happiness* most of the time when we're dealing with them, then our outlook in life, when we are in their space or they in ours, appears to lean the *most* toward the range of feeling an internal *locus of control*. This means that when we're with them we find ourselves believing that life is generally good for us and that we primarily feel that life and its circumstances fall well within our control. This will equate to a +3 as described before. On our scale of *locus of control* this is the *most* we can feel in control of our life and circumstances. If that person was a parent or guardian while we were growing up, we stand a very good chance of having developed an outlook on life that reflects a feeling of *Self-Trust and Confidence* and, consequently, with a faith in our ability to do whatever we set out to do with a minimum of interference with the outside world. So activities we share with that person will usually accentuate our sense of mostly being in charge and in control of our lives leading us to feel supported in feeling *Self-Trust and Confidence* in our ability to face the world and accomplish whatever we set out to do.

What's interesting about the people on our list, and others like them, is that if they should exit our lives and worldly space through death, moving away or just becoming out of reach through other circumstances, we would instinctively gravitate toward others with whom we can feel the same rapport and stimulation and then take steps to bring and keep them closer to us in order to fill a perceived gap in our lives. This occurs because of two reasons; first, because we felt good about ourselves when we were around them but, more importantly and much more instinctively, as humans we strive to keep a consistency and familiarity with our life patterns. So replacing their absence fulfills our *ego's* much needed sense of security, which in turn validates to us our perceived control.

In this, it's easy to see that we would always want to attempt to keep a person(s) in our space whose presence had the effect of reaffirming a sense of freedom and independence so we could keep experiencing a feeling of *happiness*. After all, feeling *happiness* reaffirms and strengthens our perception that *we* are operating from an internal *locus of control*. But what if that person enables a different feeling within us - one of helplessness or frustration? And what if we grew up with that person as our parent or guardian, how would that influence how we act? What would we then believe about ourselves? Here's where this process of pairing leading to our life choices, attitudes and beliefs can become counterproductive and even hurtful to our well-being. What if when being with a parent or guardian, or even both, we felt *anger* or *fear* for the majority of the time we were with them? What would we do then? What *could* we do to feel better? How would that affect our lives and how we handle our daily activities and expectations for long-term goals? The mechanisms for our feelings and reactions would evolve the same way, only the resultant feeling and attitude we adapt would be quite different from what might be considered to be healthy or productive for us. Yet, we would still repeat it over and over again. Let me explain.

Let's start with *anger* which is a -2 on the scale and not too far down the "feeling in control" scale but still difficult enough. Remembering that *anger* has components of *disgust* (-1) however, there is more of an urge to pursue the elimination of the tension that raises *anger* within us. Realize that feeling *anger* is an involuntary *reaction* to feeling frustrated or blocked in some way. Regardless of whether the person we spend time with is actually blocking us or not, it's more important to recognize that we *feel* blocked. When we come to this realization, we might feel assisted by using *I-Dialogue* with them so we don't polarize ourselves with and intensify the *anger*. But this is often easier said than done.

We know that feeling *angry* is almost always a *reaction* to some outside stimulus and that we need to understand that we are *answering* an outside influence with resistance, which creates internal pressure, hence, the *anger*. As we mentally process that this person *makes* us angry, we are constructing or continuing to contribute to a belief that we *don't have sufficient control of our lives or circumstances when we interact with this person*. Feeling *anger* is, essentially, feeling that *someone else* has control of the situation and our urge is to *react*.

As adults we know that for a child there are many occasions where the "blocking" of certain activities is necessary to preserve the safety and welfare of the child. But when the blocking becomes more of a reaction by the parent or more done for their convenience rather than a calculated response geared toward preserving the child's safety and wellbeing, we have a problem. Excessive blocking or authoritarianism as it is called in psychology will produce excessive *anger* in a child. In this type of disciplining the child gets the message that they are neither permitted nor capable of handling their life and circumstances on their own. This totally sabotages any potential for the child to develop *Self-Trust* or *Confidence*. This also occurs when a child is coddled or over-protected. The parent's emotional dynamic may be different for over-protection but the child's resulting *anger* is the same, except that the *anger* may be layered below the child's threshold of awareness. Hopefully, if either dynamic reflects our upbringing, we might have revealed this to ourselves through the questions in the EMOTIONAL TRAIL, list #2.

It's not enough that we've determined how the *anger* is generated. We, as children, take it a step further in concretizing the pattern of *anger*, fostering resistance before we interact with the world. If, for example, we felt rising *anger* when we were chastised by our parents about our performance, the same feeling will rise again when we, as adults, encounter chastising by our employer. What's truly unfortunate is that, as children, we learned to *expect* being chastised whenever dealing with a situation related to performance. So now we enter the same type of situation with an underlying feeling of *anger* and an *expectation* of being chastised. In that *expecting* we have already polarized our behavior *drawing* its polar opposite and fulfillment...chastising. We have recreated our childhood circumstance. We become a self-fulfilling prophesy through our expectations and behavior. *Self-Trust and Confidence* are barely even in the picture. We've given away our personal power. Since we attract who we are through the behavior we broadcast (mostly unconsciously), we become a self-fulfilling prophesy on every level by virtue of our formed beliefs about ourselves and our *expectations* of ourselves and the world. Namely, that we are neither permitted nor capable of handling our life and circumstances on our own. Participating in life this way can only maintain the belief and assumption that we have very little control over our own lives and that we are governed through an exterior *locus of control.* How could we possibly believe otherwise? The kicker about having this feeling, especially as a child, is that if it was present with our parents or guardians while we were growing up, we might not even realize that there was any other way to feel within or about ourselves. Hopefully, if there was another important person in the environment with whom we felt differently, maybe we would have potentially realized that we had other options and struggled to "reset" ourselves.

The fact that our anger is a -2 on the "feeling in control" scale leaves our *Self-Trust and Confidence* in our ability to create difference in the world severely inhibited. With our attitude of what we expect renewing itself over and over again through attracting the same people and circumstances through our projected behavior, it feels like we are almost always "behind the eight ball." The hardest part of escaping the repeating circumstances is to first realize that *we* are responsible for setting the emotional stage for attracting the continuing *expected* responses, *not* the person we are relating to. We keep creating and emitting the same learned behavior and expectations and attract either it's opposite, thereby renewing the conflict, or its similar vibration through resonating with others who are also experiencing the same responses and then commiserating, validating and intensifying the self-defeating beliefs together.

There is one other point that I would like to include relative to *Apathy*. It is much more likely that *Apathy* would manifest while spiraling *down* the scale, from +3 toward -3, than it would be working our way back *up* the scale from -3 toward +3. I believe this is so because as our requirement for dealing with a lack of control becomes more intense as we descend down the scale. Because of this increasing intensity it is much more likely to manifest in a disconnection from our feelings as the pressure grows beyond our tolerance to handle our diminishing ability to feel in control.

I have explained this emotional loop in such depth so we can see the power and the tenacious inertia with which our repetitive, and mostly unconscious, emotional cycles operate within our daily lives. I say emotional cycles rather than feeling cycles because the loop becomes closed through the pairing of the feeling, the experience and the subsequent assessment and judgment of ourselves making it a self-perpetuating trigger. We now can see how something so complete and so unconscious can rest beneath the surface of our awareness to the extent that we can actually believe that our circumstances are being dictated by the world around us. This is devastating to our *Self-Trust* and *Confidence*. What remains now is only to break the loop, bringing our unconscious contributions toward continuing the behavior to the surface of our awareness and replacing them with new experiences, or a pairing, that will refocus our behaviors, perceptions and responses in a way that will bring our personal power back under our conscious control. This brings us back to using *I-Dialogue*, the five *Simple & Easy Steps* and allowing us to assess and reprogram our behavior through our seventh step, *Cleanout the Dungeon*.

What Will They Do to Us If We Don't Comply?

Once we've determined where we are on the "feeling in control" scale with all the people we've assessed, we have to determine which ones we need removal from, which ones to reprogram and which ones we want to continue with and enhance. These decisions are no-brainers, but the removals and reprogrammables are harder to reframe within ourselves because changing anything in our usual rapport will have the tendency toward rattling our foundation and emotional security, even if that emotional security is something that keeps us feeling trapped.

The people on the plus (+) side of the scale of "feeling in control" we know we'd like to enhance and bring closer, simply due to the fact that we feel better when we are in their space. We also want to draw into our lives more people who enhance those types of feelings within us. The challenge is to remove or reprogram *our reactions* to those on the lower or minus (-) scale where our interactions augment "feeling out of control." If our interactions are compounded with a need for us to be needed, our actions in changing the relationship will be much more challenging.

In dealing with the people on the minus (-) scale we will receive one of three reactions. They will either 1.) begin to acquiesce to *I-Dialogue* and our gentle promptings (and may even seem relieved that we took the effort), 2.) remove themselves from our space or 3.) strongly "rebel" against changing their perceived stability in the context of the relationship already in place. With this third group strong reactions will validate our assessments of them and our choice to use *I-Dialogue* with them. In spite of their objections and resistance, using *I-Dialogue* will begin to create clarity for us, and maybe even for them, as to what our parts in the relationship actually are. The clarity will enable us to emotionally disconnect from their coercion enough so we can, essentially, "catch our breath" and gain a fresh perspective of where the relationship needs to come to rest if we are to continue with them.

The *Simple & Easy Steps* will begin efforts in our social avenues cultivating people and circumstances with either no or almost no pre-patterned personal contact with us, thereby, providing their non-interference and allowing a rise within us of the *Elementary Feelings* that lean toward the plus (+) side of the "feeling in control" scale. The more we can cultivate toward the plus (+) side, the more we will be able to nudge our operating *locus of control* toward feeling that we have more of an influence in our lives. With *I-Dialogue* offering more clarity and *Simple & Easy Steps* initiating new and different experiences, all we have left to do is work on step seven - *Cleanout the Dungeon.*

If you're reading this book and have gotten this far, there's a very high probability that one, if not both, of your parents or guardians provided an environment that encouraged you to feel Elementary Feelings more toward the minus (-) side than the plus (+) side of the "feeling in control" scale. And if that's the case it's also very likely that any plus (+) influences you might have felt came from people in your peripheral environment enabling you to become aware of a difference and wish that your upbringing could have gone differently. If this is the case you may have also become aware of feeling resentful of your actual parental history.

Working on parents, guardians and close friends with *I-Dialogue* and the *Small & Easy Steps* is apt to create a few stressful issues for us and those we work with. To begin with, even if what we are doing is done subtly, they will sense that something is different about us. As our activities take us more outside their space and influence, they will perceive a gap in their relationship with us. And if the relationship with them involves any obligations, expectations or dependencies - and with family and close friends it usually does - they will begin to recognize the absence of what they need in the relationship and accusations of our being selfish may come to the surface. This will come as no surprise to many of us. Odds are we've felt its pressure many times before when we've attempted to venture out on our own. Normally, when we feel a familiar person or situation slipping out of our space, our reaction is to grasp or hold them tighter in order to preserve our sense of consistency and security with them. We are creatures of habit. When a consistent rapport changes, we feel it, sometimes unconsciously, and we still react. So as we progress in weaning ourselves from entangling emotional interactions it's best to be prepared for some "push-back" because we'll undoubtedly receive some. As we do, it is of the utmost importance that we hold our emotional "repositioning" long enough that our parent or close friend is able to acclimate to the changes. Simply put, it's like breaking in a new pair of shoes. At first they are uncomfortable and draw our attention but, eventually, we get used to the feel and we soon forget about the change as we're distracted by other circumstances. This will result as a consequence of implementing both *I-Dialogue* the *Simple & Easy Steps*. If we are consistent and persistent enough, we may even begin to nudge *them* up on the "feeling in control" scale and our frequency of feeling their influence on the minus (-) scale will diminish. Be aware though that they may either intensify the pressure on us and/or they could simply attempt to get what they need from another family member. You must also remember that the other family member's emotional state of being *is not your responsibility*. They must, at some point, learn to do what you are doing if they are to free themselves from their own limiting behavior. If the pressure on us increases, and it most likely will, so must our resolve. Remember, we are in control of how *we* behave. No one can *make* us do anything. We always have the ability to choose even in the direst of circumstances.

There is a subtle understanding which needs to be surfaced here. First, when we are working with someone who is operating on a level that is feeling more out of control than we are, that is, working more in the (-) *Elementary Feelings* scale than the (+) side of "feeling in control," there is a tendency for their *ego* to resist our change of focus in order to justify, to themselves, that their *ego* is still in control even at the expense of living within limits that are self-hurtful. In this case their security and validation of their *projection* is more important to them than any potential for personal accomplishment available through altering their life approach. When we interact with others their natural instinct, and usually ours, is to keep or bring the conversation to subjects that *they* find of interest, safe from the exposure of their perceived inadequacies, and that agree with their current self-assessment and projected image. What this means to us is that their urge to pull us into *their* world of beliefs and perspectives, thereby solidifying and protecting their validation of their self-image and insuring their ego's survival feels much stronger than their desire for inner growth. In this light we have to understand that we will arrive at a point where we will have to make a decision whether our interaction with them can be reprogrammed to operate more on the (+) scale of "feeling in control" thereby supporting our new emotional "repositioning," rather than (-) where must we "cut them loose" to prevent our "going down with the ship" through participating in commiseration. This decision can be *extremely* difficult while currently still loving them, especially after having originally believed that we must remain loyal to our prior emotional history in supporting them while they supported us.

And that word would be – don't. Unless you are working with another person who is also doing this work, you can expect little or no support from anyone else. What you are doing through these steps is reprogramming your responses to the efforts and expectations of others. You must remember that you are not only responding to the early reprogramming provided by your family and those close to you but also social expectations which will not be as supportive as what you might expect.

In the face of our Western culture's apparent and ardent surface emphasis on healing and rebalancing ourselves and the compassion expected for those of us who need assistance in reclaiming health, there exists a subliminal assumption and negative judgment by our society about the methods we use for that same recovery.

The methods utilized for most of us feeling on the (-) minus scale of *Elementary Feelings* and wishing to move toward the (+) side of our feelings that reflect a more internal *locus of control* often do not meet with the approval of social expectations or demands. Our use of them appears to fall under a double standard of labeling. On the one hand, our emotional difficulties fall under the social label of needing and deserving social assistance, yet our methods for healing ourselves are tacitly labeled as being, essentially selfish and anti-social. Let me provide some brief examples.

Fear and its sister feelings, *depression and helplessness*, are well known for presenting an appearance of its most obvious of induced symptoms, immobilization. Medication may reduce our sensitivity to or awareness of having these feelings but do nothing to eradicate their cause. That immobilization can be seen as the stagnation or blocking of our energy. With no energy, there is no movement. We feel trapped, depressed and stuck with no apparent way for us to feel better. One of our most potent motivators is *anger* – the next *Elementary Feeling* (-2) on the emotional scale. It is our most powerful agitant toward leaving a field of immobility. It is almost always *anger* that is responsible for moving us from the immobilization of *depression, fear* and *helplessness* to a freer more mobile condition in life. But there is a problem. Our culture and social standards label *anger* as an inappropriate and unacceptable avenue for interacting with others. *Anger* further viewed as being selfish and its application is seen as an imposition on others. What are we to do? On the one hand society condones our movement and efforts toward health and well-being yet, condemns our most effective means for finding relief.

Moving up through the other *Elementary Feelings* on the emotional scale also meets similar oppositions through double standard labeling. Moving from *anger* (-2) toward *disgust* (-1) utilizes an exchange from the need to act prevalent in *anger* with simply letting go of what we're angry about and relegating it to an assessment of preference leading to our acceptance or rejection of the people and circumstances involved. However, our culture sees our acceptance or rejection of others as being egotistical – another inappropriate and unacceptable behavior.

In moving from *disgust* (-1) toward *sadness* (+1) we utilize *sadness* in releasing our feelings of *disgust* through simply allowing ourselves to feel the *sadness*. But again, this behavior is seen as inappropriate and unacceptable and deemed an imposition on the moods of others and to be pitied in public but ostracized and avoided in private. This label addresses our culturally elicited guilt for not being our brother's keeper and for our responsibility for showing compassion through relieving someone else's problems.

In moving from *sadness* (+1) toward *surprise* (+2) we utilize *surprise* in moving from feeling bad for someone else's difficulties toward not allowing another's circumstances to have an affect us. Our culture views this behavior as lacking compassion.

You might think, "What possible negative label could be applied when moving from *surprise* (+2) toward *happiness* (+3)?" The answer is - none. The move from *surprise* toward *happiness* is relatively negligible as we expect circumstances to be more in line with our desires and free of surprises. Our culture applies no derogatory labels to *happiness* since it is a culturally professed objective. However, for many, jealousy becomes a very strong undercurrent with a conflicting wish to avoid acknowledging someone else's feeling happy while at the same time wishing to move into their space in the hopes that some of the feeling may "rub off" on us.

My purpose in bringing these perspectives to the surface is not to promote or develop pessimism but to make us all aware that there are many dynamics operating within our social constructs that contradict one another. The most important understanding to take away from this perspective is that expecting support for our moving up the emotional scale is not likely if not impossible. This is a task we must tackle alone.

We are all creatures of habit and as such we may not have the emotional strength *at the time* to "push through" the pressure levied on us, coercing our resumption of the comfortable, yet restrictive, emotional structure our parents and guardians have created for us. As in meditation, when we realize that we have slipped from our chosen path, it's extremely important that we don't beat ourselves up for not gaining the reactions from others that we desire. Feeling and behaving this way will only serve to reinforce the diminished *Self-Trust and Confidence* we felt in the first place. Simply acknowledge the slippage, pick yourself up, dust yourself off, and resume the journey. Like any skill, it takes time to develop proficiency and a consistent and recognizable pattern that we can then continually reinforce and strengthen through repetitively resuming our new emotional "repositioning." It took many years throughout our childhood to create this pattern. It will not change overnight. As we create more emotional space for ourselves, just like in the forest example, the new pattern, through continued reapplication and reinforcement, will gain enough momentum to produce a state of inertia, just like it did when we were children, which will eventually become strong enough to carry us toward feeling what we choose to feel.

SELF-TRUST & MOTIVATION:
The Eternal Dance

From a Layman's Perspective

Our Preliminary Understandings

There were many things that I wanted to do and be when I was growing up. Yet, as an adult, they never manifested. When I tried, I almost always ended up feeling discouraged and deflated. It seemed like I always met insurmountable resistance to my efforts. My reaction was to attribute that resistance to external circumstances, competition, and other people and, sometimes, just plain bad luck. It took many years to realize that the resistance that I felt was actually my own. When I did realize and accept it, I was puzzled as to where within me it had come from. Anytime I reached out past my familiar envelope resistance was there waiting like a shark beneath the surface of the ocean. There began a long process of reading, self-help books and classes, therapy and a holy host of other self-improvement gimmicks and methods for "personal success" plunging me into the field of psychology and metaphysics in a desperate attempt to gnaw away at the pillars of self-doubt and self-worth standing in the way of my feeling like a whole person.

To confuse the issue, in some areas of my life I would shine and be a beacon of talent and accomplishment. In others, I would fail so miserably that I wanted to slink away into the nearest cave and hide out in shame. How could I feel so adept in one area in my life and so completely inadequate in another?

It seemed irrational to me. In my journeys through psychology I learned about the unconscious. I had found another scapegoat to account for the resistance I now know and had to accept as having originated within me. The key to the validation of this was that I was told, and believed, that my unconscious was out of my control; I was not responsible. When I struggled against my own fears, I became a self-fulfilling prophesy. This only served to verify that my inability was "not my fault." If no fault insurance has taught us anything, it's taught us that everything is a two way street…it takes two to tango. Little did I know that in struggling with the fear I was simply holding on to it and that doing so only served to increase its power over me. Learning *Law of Attraction* principles has only recently confirmed that understanding within me. Additionally, there's a Chinese proverb in the martial arts that states "to acknowledge your enemy gives them power over you." In focusing on my fears, I was doing just that - giving them the power to strengthen the resistance within me. In comprehending and absorbing this I began to get a handle on the key as to what held my fears and inadequacies in place. My mind began to understand the dynamics but I was a long way from dealing with, let alone understanding, the feelings that were coupled with my entrenched resistance. Instinctively, I knew that there was a "switch" somewhere in my makeup that could enable me to turn this around and I was determined to find it and throw it. But how deep and how far would I have to go to gain access and have control? I didn't know but I was sure willing to work toward it. Anything was better than the pain of resistance and immobility.

Every action we take, or don't, in the physical world is governed by a choice. Either we go or we don't. Either we get married or we don't. Either we steal or we don't. Either we go to sleep or stay up. The world is filled with "polarized" choices.

Sometimes we make these choices while we're unaware of them and while we're involved with larger and more pressing matters. In these cases they occur below the threshold of our awareness. The key toward understanding them is that every choice and action we take or not is *still* within our control. We may have many reasons or excuses why we do or don't do something but the bottom line is that it always comes back to us and our choices. Yes, others in the world *do* have an influence over what choices we make. But we let them. In the long run, and if we're honest with ourselves, we have to admit that the responsibility for our *choices* and *actions does* rest solely with us. It's the *consequences* that we are only *half* responsible for since we have no play over the choices and actions *others* make and take in situations in which we both participate. We must remember that relating with others is *always* a two way street. We can't blame anyone else for *our* choices or actions.

So how, then, is it that we allow ourselves to feel so coerced, so inhibited, so encouraged, so enabled by an invisible yet powerful urge to take this direction over that? What is it within us that is so powerful and so effective in urging us to make the same choices over and over and over again?

This urge, this motivation, this causality for our choices is established at birth or soon after. But, you say, at that age how can we even think or rationalize a choice? We don't even have a language with which to do it. But if you go deep inside, past the language, past the thinking, past the senses of your body, you know that there is something within you that is much more encompassing than just these things. It's our feelings. And our feelings are innate and triggered by our experiences. If we are nurtured by someone, we feel love. If we are ignored or treated badly by someone we feel fear. The key to understanding this is that in the physical world *every experience* we encounter elicits a reaction, a feeling, within us. This reaction, this feeling is a *shared* experience. It is part of our interrelation with others. Remember it takes two to tango? This is no different. These feelings are elicited with every encounter we have with another person, every reaction to what we experience in the world. However, feelings are *not* within our control. They simply occur. It is *these* reactions and feelings that present the basis for every other choice that we make throughout our lives and it is only *those choices* that we have control over. Please understand that feelings are *not* emotions. There is a dramatic difference between them, which I will cover and explain and re-emphasize throughout this book. Feelings are only one of the components contained *within* emotion. For now, please just accept that feelings occur in the moment and that they are entities unto themselves. With all this in mind let's examine the new developing landscape that provides the basis for our choices.

Where Do We Start?

Bear with me here. This will seem rather long and convoluted but will give you an understanding of where our ability and *willingness* to act come from, how early they develop and why they may be so difficult to activate. It's important to note that the trigger for our willingness comes from our feelings. It is *extremely* important to understand that learning language and developing the mind *completely* changes our perspective on how we *deal* with our feelings. Our culture has become so obsessed with the mind and its performance that we have lost most of our awareness of and connection to our feelings and our ability to deal with them. What follows is an explanation of the process of how this occurs. When you read this, please be in a place where you can concentrate, undisturbed and focus clearly on recognizing the underlying concepts. You may have to read through once or twice to get the feel of what I'm putting forward. The prior section has explained what we can do to counteract these influences.

The first thing that needs to be understood is *motivation* and what it really is. Everyone might have a different idea about this so it will be best if I give you a dictionary meaning so we're on the same page. *Motivation* is a derivative of the word *move* which comes from the Latin *movere* meaning 'to move, set in motion, remove or disturb' (etymonline.com). So, it's whatever impels us into action or movement. Now, we all understand things that can encourage our interest or catch our attention toward a subject, circumstance or activity. What most of us don't realize is that the "power switch" or the "go-button" that actually allows us to get moving is almost always solely dependent on our *Self-Trust and Confidence* in our ability to manage what is needed to handle that movement. If we lack *Self-Trust and Confidence* or if they are diminished in any way, action most likely won't happen.

The next questions that beg to be asked are Where do *Self-Trust and Confidence* come from and what are they? Are they learned? Inherited? Given? In answer, we might say all three since they develop during our early formative years through the interaction between us and our caretakers. They are qualities that start developing within us *before* we develop language skills. You might say, "Well, that's sort of vague," and you'd be right, because at that age our language skills have yet to be developed and *all* our interactions occur in the feeling mode. To learn, inherit or receive, which are qualities of exchange, implies that they come partly from our relationship with our environment. But becoming aware or sensing how we separate into the environment soon after birth is a newly occurring experience and we have also not yet formed an awareness of that separation let alone how to navigate it. Because we are humans and the quality of separation has been fairly well developed in most of us as adults it may be difficult for us to identify with this state of "no mind." A baby, initially, exists in this state of no mind, or in a "soup" of feeling. This is one of the reasons we adult humans find it so difficult to move into meditation and free ourselves from the discriminating, gymnastic and pervasive mind. It's hard for us to get back into a much earlier empty state that we no longer remember. So, as a child, this pre-verbal or pre-mind state is just beginning to develop our awareness of separation. In this polarized environment our newly and slowly developing mind *IS* a vehicle of separation. As a baby, our only interactions with the world consist of involuntary body functions, crying and laughing and how we connect them to our feelings.

So, we still don't know what *Self-Trust and Confidence* are, but we're well on our way toward understanding their genesis.

As babies, laughing and crying are almost always a reaction to what we feel in the moment *and* a response to what we're feeling coming from our caretakers as tangible or intangible as that may be. When we're born we emerge from a self-sustaining (mother generated) environment into a world of polarity where we must interact with others for support. It's difficult enough to deal with the separation that comes with being born, but it's even more intense to have no sense of or experience in navigating within that separation since we've emerged from a world where everything has been previously provided for. Birth truly is a traumatic experience. This focus on navigation heightens our need to develop an *external* awareness and focus.

In that external focus the first thing we feel *outside* of our *own* feelings are our caretakers' responses, or lack of the same, to our laughing or crying. Here we begin to make the connection between our action and the outside world but *only through our feelings*. Remember, we have no language or thinking skills developed yet and it's still all about what we're feeling. If the responses we receive from our caretakers are in line with our support and what we need, we "pair" our feeling and action with their response and begin a rudimentary memory of their responses within our feelings. It's almost like we're creating new instincts. In receiving what we need, we can say that our developing and socializing might allow a normalcy to occur, relative to where we pay attention and, as yet, producing no appreciable difference between internal or external. If, however, we perceive that our quest for support is ignored or met with resistance, or apathy by our caretakers, we develop a feeling or instinct of lack and our attitude becomes much more concentrated on things external as a result of the intensity of the augmented need we now feel. As we grow in our ability to distinguish between ourselves and others, our attitude or instinct concerning what we have or haven't received begins to form a hazy set of fundamental building blocks for developing a feeling of worth. If we've received what we need physically and emotionally, that is, food, safety, comfort, touch and good attention, that attitude will enable a balance of attention between us and our external world. In the case of not receiving what we need, our attention migrates more toward a feeling or instinct of lack, while strengthening its connection to the external and the fact that lack is somehow connected to the responses of others to our expression (laughing or crying). The balance between our internal and external attention then becomes distorted more toward external and we begin losing attentiveness to our *own* internal feelings in anticipation of needed external worldly responses. Our developing sense of separation is still occurring through this interaction but in a slower and more lopsided way.

At this point you're probably asking yourself ,Why would I care where my attention goes? The point is that where our attention goes, hence our energy, is where our initial experiences in development take place. Those experiences set the first foundations forming our attitude in facing the world. If we don't receive a response, or at least a preferred response, to our efforts and quest for support our exertions (laughing and crying) in those directions will slowly diminish but our attention to the feeling of lack will remain. As with any conditioning or encouragement, lack of reward diminishes behavior but not necessarily attention.

Remember, as a child our mind and ability to separate, let alone put what we feel into words, has only *begun* to form. We still live well within the undifferentiated soup of feeling, partly hanging between our own feelings and partly through empathizing what our caretakers feel. When the mind is not in control, or almost entirely absent, we are left with only our feelings and empathy – our inner sea of diffusion with minimal-separation. This may be difficult for us to comprehend given that we have lived the major part of our lives in the separative, time constricted environment of our minds…so much so that some of us think that we *are* our minds.

So, we now can see that our initial memories and reactions to our first attempts to receive the support and nurturance that we need (through laughing or crying) occur in a non-verbal or pre-verbal mode within the realm of our feelings or instincts. It's important to note here that learning the language and developing the mind not only creates a separation between the things we identify and recognize but distance and separation is *also created between our feelings and our mind*. When you're thinking *about* something you're no longer in the moment feeling it. This means that what is felt pre-verbally is total in its intensity making *all* our first memories powerfully encompassing and nebulous through our feelings. Learning the language and developing the mind separates us from our feelings making it much harder to deal with the "pairing" or memories made pre-verbally, let alone describing them.

Secondly, it's also important to note that if we *don't* get the support we seek, our attention becomes more fixated on what's happening *externally* than *internally* or on the needed balance between them. This early *external* focus on receiving negative responses is the crux of our tendency to short circuit motivation which, you will remember, is powered by our *Self-Trust and Confidence* in receiving what we want or need through our efforts. That *Self-Trust* and *Confidence*, essentially, equates to a learned expectation or faith in our ability based on our pre-verbal experiences. Because these responses occur during our pre-verbal stage it is virtually impossible to effect a change in our *Self-Trust and Confidence* using affirmations, skill improvement, peer encouragement or monetary incentives (contrived mental transcripts) in the face of *feeling* or "knowing" that we will expect negative responses. These "tricks" simply give attention to what we feel we *can't* do and add energy and momentum to its influence. This is so because the earlier feelings established through the creation of our pre-verbal memory have not been altered by them relative to our previously learned expectations. Language and mind are only *tools*. Feeling is an *experience*. To change our *expectations*, which control whether we act or not, we must change our *feelings* by creating new experiences that support our *Self-Trust and Confidence* in our ability to be effective in our actions. This statement is extremely important to understand and digest so I will repeat it. To change our *expectations*, which control whether we act or not, we must change our *feelings* by creating new experiences that support our *Self-Trust and Confidence* in our ability to be effective in our actions.

So the factors that contribute the most toward acting on our motivations are our feelings, pre- and post-verbal, the type and amount of support and nurturance we've pre-verbally received, the degree to which we focus externally as opposed to internally and our expectations relative to all the other factors. Our internal/external relationship with our environment holds a lot more bearing than you might think and has a very profound effect on whether we develop as an introvert or extravert. This will become clearer as we broaden our understanding of our internal/external relationship with the world.

The Destructive Power of "Constructive" Criticism

When we begin a new project or we make an important decision in our culture we tend to ask for feedback from the people we love and respect. Sometimes we even ask for feedback from those we might consider as an adversary and even sometimes those we fear. Yet, we maintain our awareness and defensiveness with them. The most common place where we usually receive the most undermining influences are from those we love and respect because when we relate to them we are more likely to blindly take to heart what they say due to our trust in them. Hence, we are less likely to be diligent in discriminating their feedback as fully as those we might consider to be adversaries.   What may be difficult for us to consider is that even though those we love and respect may have good intentions, their responses may be more in line with their *own* agendas relative to their *own* emotional or social survival, which may not necessarily gel with what we're looking for from their feedback. In that case the feedback may do more harm than good by discouraging what we intend rather than offering the support we might desire or even expect from them.

In assessing our feedback we have two factors to consider: first, how strong is the *Self-Trust and Confidence* we feel in what we're asking about and its effect on our propensity to ask for feedback and, second, what in *their* agendas might interfere with *our* motivations? Let's first look at our own *Self-Trust* and *Confidence.*

As a general rule, most people ask for feedback regardless of their degree of *Self-Trust* and *Confidence.* However, the lower the degree possessed the more likely we will be to ask for feedback and follow suggestions with little or no personal discrimination. If we align with an external *locus of control,* that is, have learned to more likely follow what occurs *outside* of ourselves as we were trained to do in childhood, we will, additionally, tend to take to heart and follow blindly any external feedback we receive. If we have aligned with an internal *locus of control,* that is, we were trained in childhood to trust our *own* judgment, we will examine the feedback more closely and be less likely to blindly do or follow whatever we've been told. To better understand *locus of control* and its relevancy to *motivation,* please read the article *"The Importance of Internal & External Attention"* in the *Layman's Perspective* section.

There are, obviously, many points of balance between the extremes of our internal and external attentiveness with many mixtures of varying proportion. That balance, or imbalance, can also shift when different issues are dealt with or when a different person is consulted. So as our *Self-Trust and Confidence* level varies between people and issues, our choice to act or not will also vary. We may act in some situations and not in others. However, the lower the degree of *Self-Trust and Confidence* we have, which is when we listen more to what we're told than what we feel, the less likely we will be to act on our *motivations.* This brings us to the agendas of the people we are asking for that feedback.

It is my chosen, and experienced, belief that *no one* does anything for purely one reason. We have to admit that when we decide to do something it is *always* because the potential outcome of the plan chosen offers more options for success than the other choices available. That is, it satisfies more than one wish, need or requirement. So it is with everyone. Most everyone chooses their actions based on the best all-around potential. If the choice includes helping another or ending up in a "good light" as one of the potential outcomes we are more than likely going to choose that option(s). We must recognize and remember that we are all still half animal and that half has an inborn selfish perspective geared toward survival, if not dominance...physically and emotionally. The fact that many of us attempt to deny that fact or are simply unconscious of it is only testimony to the fact that our survival options almost always remain unconsciously cloaked by more altruistic ones. For example, we may assist a family member with some task in their home because it allows us access to the good looking neighbor that just moved in next to them. We can choose to be altruistic in our explanations but still harbor a hidden agenda relative to our animal side. It's those cloaked agendas that I want to draw your attention to.

The first is *self-doubt*. If the person we ask for feedback is too afraid to do something, they may emphatically recommend that *we* take that action to see if there is the potential for a successful outcome. Hence, *we* take the risk. For example, if we are at work in an office and we ask another for advice about asking for a raise, they may be more inclined to encourage us to do so in order to see if the field is clear for them to ask also. If we get shot down, they've avoided the risk and remain in a positive light with the boss. Not so for us.

The second agenda is the power of *feeling in control*. If the person we ask for advice feels insignificant or feels out of control in *their lives*, they may simply tell us to act in a way that we ordinarily wouldn't just to feel their own power, even if the recommended action sabotages our advantage in doing what we're asking about. This may also make them feel like we were asking for their permission to act. This agenda is also getting us to *give them our power*. For example, if we were to ask someone about going back to school in order to get qualified to acquire and do a specific job, they may tell us all the bad things about going back to school like paying for it, having to use our leisure time to study, the commuting we'd have to do and a whole host of other reasons, all the while believing that an education may be the best thing for *us*. The added bonus for them is being able to rationalize not feeling self-conscious about *not* making the effort *themselves*.

The third agenda is ***jealousy***. If the person we ask for advice feels that we have an innate skill that they don't but wish they had themselves, they may advise us to act in a way that would lead us toward losing or ignoring that skill by squandering it. For example, if we are good at sports and the person we asked is not, but would like to be and is jealous of our ability, they might advise us to turn down a scholarship or redirect us into a field which doesn't utilize our skills. They may then appease their guilt by telling themselves that their advice was more practical and less of a gamble than our risk of "not making the team."

The last agenda I want to speak about is the ***transfer of limitations***. This will probably be one of the more common methods of thwarting our *motivation* and will most likely be an unconscious sabotage by the person we ask. The person may support the action about which we're asking advice but may offer methods that may inhibit or interfere with what our intentions are. For example, if we are asking for directions on how to get somewhere, someone may tell us the usual way that *they* get there. In using their way we may find much more traffic than we would have encountered had we taken a path provided by *our own* intuition. In other words, other people's ways and paths for doing things may not gel with the ways that would be easiest for us. In the long run they may slow us down or altogether halt our progress.

These are just a few examples of others' agendas that may interfere with our acting on activities that we've been garnering momentum to partake in. Some agendas are rational and some may be irrational but the effect on our choice to act will be the same. The truth about most of these agendas that act like saboteurs is that they are most often done by people *unconsciously*. That is, they don't realize consciously that what they are telling us to do is more advantageous to *them* and in line with what *they* want than us. This means that any accusations made on our part could really end us up in hot water with the people we ask since they are *not aware* of their unconscious agendas themselves.

So what is the best path? If we *have to* ask for advice, we must do our due diligence in personally discriminating the advice we receive from others. Their intentions may consciously be in a good place but their unconscious needs and wants may get the better of them and in *our* way. Remember, the stronger our *Self-Trust and Confidence* are, the less need we will have to ask for advice or feedback and the less likely we will be to follow it without due diligence. We must work on our own *Self-Trust and Confidence* first. Then our choices will reflect more clearly what our spirit intends.

The Importance of Internal & External Attention

Whether we focus internally or externally contributes a tremendous amount of influence to what we come to believe about ourselves and how we expect life to progress. Let me show you the connections.

When we *don't* receive the responses or nurturance that we need or want from our caretakers, we are trained into focusing *outside* of ourselves more than paying attention to what we feel within. This is because our *feeling* for a lack of nurturance seems to us to be a nebulous parental resistance and intensifies our feeling of yearning leading us to focus on and intensify our sensitivity to what is external in the anticipation of our desired response from them. In this interchange the majority of our focus has shifted to what is external through our yearning for that response. Through this experience and others that are similar we form instincts and expectations for future responses. Our inner feelings then become relegated to participating as a trigger for our future external expectations. It appears to be a felt and perceived lack that produces a polarity and draws our attention toward what is external. It is satiation that allows it to remain internal and free of polarizing influences. On other words, when we have no needs, we tend not to focus outside of ourselves. An example of this is when we are *in utero*.

This whole process occurs pre-verbally. Later and post-verbally the mind will begin to develop language and thought leading to "morphing" those expectations into beliefs about our world (a belief is just a thought that we keep thinking). Thus begins our rudimentary pre-verbal expectation and post-verbal belief that our world is controlled by external forces and circumstances. This happens as a continual process cascading its effects throughout our lives but most strongly beginning from birth to age five. In psychological terms it is the developing of this externally directed perception of and attitude toward life that is labeled external *locus of control*. In its extreme form this is the belief that all choices, all circumstances and all our needs and wants are determined by others and that we have no power of our own. The acceptance of this creates a partnership of perspectives. First, that we have no active part in what we will receive or what happens around us. This, as our developing mind begins to form a basic acclimation toward it, facilitates a very small jump toward justifying and projecting blame for our circumstances on those external to us if those circumstances become unpleasant and/or unwanted. Second, this perspective eliminates the possibility of developing any semblance of accountability for those circumstances. Conversely, the developed belief (remember, a belief is just a thought we keep thinking) that others wield all the power over our lives creates the perception that there is something missing or wrong with us. When we begin with this feeling and mental assertion of perceived inadequacy, we spend the rest of our lives attempting to compensate for that lack by employing social *defense mechanisms* to assign blame and cloak the fact that we feel inadequate. This is in alignment with Alfred Adler's theory that we *all* start life with an initial *inferiority complex* due to the fact that as newborns and babies we *must* be dependent on our caretakers for our initial support until we are able to fend for ourselves. They and all they are connected to are viewed as Omni-powerful. When *Self-Trust and Confidence* are subsequently *not* developed through learning to make our own choices, or being allowed to do so, that *inferiority complex* expands and continues through life in a cloaked form.

At this point it's important to note that it is believed by many professionals that all newborns, babies and young children start life with an instinct or feeling that they are inferior to the power of their caretakers and other outsiders due to their inability to satisfy their own needs. Obviously, without the mind being developed this is a very elusive perspective for us to contemplate. Perhaps, as adults, the closest we can compare this nebulous feeling to is intimidation. Ironically, and as a civilization we *still* don't know what instincts or feelings actually are or where they come from. All we know is that they exist, are essentially involuntary and that we feel them. The point I'm moving toward here is that if our caretakers *do not* endeavor to begin allowing us, as children, to develop preferences, as simple as those choices may be, we will continue to *feel* that we have no effect on satisfying our own needs or determining our own circumstances and conditions and will continue to focus *outside* ourselves for direction and permission. Currently, a *very* small part of our population focuses on teaching us to build trust in ourselves by allowing us to express preferences. This allowing gives us the feeling that we have *some* power over our conditions and begins to develop a rudimentary *Self-Trust* and *Confidence* within us. It's important to note that it's not that the majority of parents and caretakers don't wish to attend us through our training; it's just that many of them are not aware that it is *necessary* for the development of our *Self-Trust* and *Confidence.* Additionally, through dealing with the support of their family, career obligations, daily chores and requirements of survival, self-maintenance, and financial matters there are created such overwhelming stresses and demands that parents and caretakers often just don't have the energy to observe or perceive clearly our emotional needs, or to invest in what is inwardly necessary for our growth toward independent support. There are so many external demands that now draw us all toward the tangible world that many of us no longer have the opportunity to invest in our *own* emotional needs and well-being let alone knowing what is necessary for our children. To wit, how many times have we observed a parent asking a child what they think or feel? It doesn't occur very frequently with most of us.

Our culture has become so material and so excessively outer directed that it is hard to recognize the need to "go inside" and attend our *own* feelings. If we don't do it with ourselves, how can we guide our children to do so? The few of us that *are* trained and allowed to express preferences in childhood grow into having a sense that we are able to have *some* effect on our own well-being, if not our environment. In *having this experience* we develop *Self-Trust and Confidence* in ourselves. As we grow into adults we come to feel and believe that we *can*, generally, control our own life and conditions. Psychologists call this having an internal *locus of control*; that is, that our life path and circumstances are mostly directed and controlled *by our own actions*. We, as these types of children, often grow up to become the most effective leaders, pioneers and world changers.

Although it is not possible to second guess all of our child's needs and requirements, especially as pre-verbal babies, we *do* have the ability to take time and observe how they interact with the world and can generally figure out where to apply support so they can develop *Self-Trust and Confidence* in their ability to deal with the world, at the least partially, on their own terms. Most of us who don't know what we want out of life are usually the children who were never given the opportunity to think about our preferences and who were simply pressed into just following the social expectations that we were issued. Listening to our children has become a lost art and a sorely needed activity. Not having the time or energy is a poor excuse at best. For us as adults, even now, to feel *Self-Trust and Confidence* we *must have* the types of experiences and reinforcements that lead us toward developing them. Sadly, many of us have not had external reinforcement leading to those types of experiences in our childhood. But it is never too late for us to put them into place ourselves with our creativity and a little selfishness. Yes, I said selfishness...that tremendous social taboo.

So far I've spoken about what we're left with from our journey through our pre-verbal period of childhood. In review: If we *haven't* received the nurturance and attention that we need or require during our pre-verbal period we are left with a feeling of emptiness or lack, a heightened focus on the external world and a diminished focus on our inner world. This makes us lean more in the direction of an exterior *locus of control* or toward the feeling that our life circumstances are controlled almost solely by forces external to us. If we *have* received most of the nurturance and attention that we need or require during our pre-verbal period, which is not as likely as it might seem, our feeling of emptiness or lack will be much less, leaning us more toward a balance between internal and external *locus of control* and the feeling that our life circumstances are controlled almost equally between our efforts and the outside world, but with a small degree more toward external (this is resonant with Adler's *inferiority complex*). In dealing with only our feelings, this seems to be a fairly clear distinction between perspectives. But when we add the developing working of the mind, or slowly shift away from our pre-verbal phase and gradually into the verbal phase, a curious thing happens. We begin making rational memories of our new cascading experiences and then our pre-verbal experiences become overshadowed by the new and usable clarity of our verbal development. This enhances and then solidifies our ability to rationalize our circumstances based on external factors.

It's difficult enough not receiving the attention and the support we need to develop our *Self-Trust and Confidence*, but furthering our understanding of our *inferiority complex* to a degree, *past* our simple feelings of pre-verbal lack and unanswered needs opens us up to a new avenue for personal diminishment *and/or* improvement. This occurs during and through the acquisition of language and our thinking skills. Our sense of time, language and thinking develop in codependent partnership with each other. Each pair needs the third member for its definition and discrimination. They are completely interwoven and interdependent. The mind and language work together by the principle of separation, which is enabled through learning and utilizing the concept of past, present and future. This may seem difficult for some of us to comprehend, but suffice it to say that as these three develop together our nebulous and undefined pre-verbal experiences slowly fade into our subconscious. As they do so, those experiences become virtually unreachable due to the fact that they've never had thoughts attached to them. So, during this time there is a major shift in our perception *and* a window of time where adjusted verbal reinforcement through a new parental perspective and involvement *might* compensate for any previous lost nurturance or attention affecting our growing *Self-Trust* and *Confidence*.

Being drawn into the physical world was just the first step in beginning to distance ourselves from what we're feeling and simply reacting to. Now we begin to use a tool that adds structure to that distancing by talking *about* our experiences and feelings. Remember, when we talk *about* what we're feeling we're no longer aware of *having* the experience of feeling. We're distancing ourselves from it. But at this point you might say, "But, isn't it good to be able to talk about our feelings?" and I would say yes, it is, but it's also good to be able to compare and discuss those feelings with another person. Why? Because having the ability to deal with them *mentally* enables us to prevent being swept away by them…at least for the moment. The key to the mind's potential and effectiveness is in detaching us from our feelings so that it enables us to pull away from solely *reacting* to them. Think about it. If you're no longer having a feeling there is less possibility for you to simply and "mindlessly" react to it. This doesn't *eliminate* our feelings. It just enables us to *refocus* on something else. That something else is literally another *head space* that allows us to see a bigger and more rational picture. This is the essence of our growing awareness. Remember, we begin as spirit. Being born into a physical body is a traumatic experience, removing us from our safe and self-contained environment. Our birth now adds or incorporates an animal nature into our larger "self." In developing our mind and its language we are providing a means of mediating the "heaven and earth" and "spirit and matter" that we have paired together by being born. This merging often takes a lifetime just to learn to be able to navigate through. Both body and spirit have their own "urges" and our lives are, essentially, a battle over which one has dominance. The key is that we must "grow them" to work together. The mind is an intermediary and a tool that can facilitate that goal.

In learning a language you might say that it will put us all on the same page when it comes to having meaning. That may be true but only partially so. Where it's true is where it aligns with dictionary meanings, contemporary social traditions and expectations. Where it will be different is where it is attached to each of our individual and personal experiences. For example, the first day of school will be a different experience for each of us. So when we are asked about school we each will have a different way of describing it depending on what we've done and experienced. In the same vein of difference, and what is not as obvious, is that we will each have one or a combination of a small number of *Elementary Feelings* (no pun intended)also attached to the experience. From a different perspective, and since different experiences can be "paired" with the *same* feelings, our feelings will be *described differently* for each of us as language is absorbed and incorporated into our awareness.

Some feelings may be described with slight differences and others may be described with radical differences. Recognizing this is an important component of compassion. The feelings that move through us are few in number but universal. How we describe them is not. Awareness for recognizing these few and *Elementary Feelings* has been researched and documented by Dr. Paul Ekman (Ekman, 2003). There are only six universal human feelings: *surprise, fear, disgust, anger, happiness and sadness*. All feelings occur *involuntarily*. Yes, I said *involuntarily*. They occur spontaneously, like a wave moving through the ocean. We have no control over the *movement* of them but we do have control over *which* ones we perceive through changing our thoughts and, thereby, *inducing* the movement of an alternate feeling. We also generally have a choice as to whether they're expressed in public. When they are *not* projected openly, whether due to our defensiveness, an intentional cloaking or self-consciousness, they can still be recognized through *micro-expressions* or through short bursts. *Micro-expressions* are fleeting facial expressions of our feelings that are projected *involuntarily* and for only one fifth of a second before our desired facial expressions are returned to what our mind says are appropriate for our experience in the current situation. The *micro-expressions* occur because the arising and movement of our feelings are *involuntary*. They "leak" through our persona. Once "flashed," the mind quickly recovers control and returns to our preferred or expected expression. We can train ourselves not to *show* our feelings but we *cannot avoid having them*. The key to managing them lies with our acquired tool, the mind. When our thinking becomes involved, the opportunity for forming *emotions* is created. Now you're probably saying to yourself, "Feeling…emotion…aren't they the same thing?" The answer is no. Let me explain why.

After physical senses, our first domain of inner movement is feelings. They occur spontaneously and like a wave. When they occur with an experience pre-verbally they are "paired" and stored as a rudimentary memory in the form of an "instinct." As a pre-verbal child there is no capacity to describe it, let alone, share it with anyone else. As we learn language and begin to form the mind, our second inner domain, new language is substituted for the instinct and the pairing and becomes much more controllable and accessible for change, through the mind and its thoughts. The vocabulary that is attributed or paired with each feeling allows the potential for us to re-experience the feeling through repeating the thought and verbal trigger. This pairing of a feeling with a thought is called *emotion*. *Emotions* are our internally generated repetitive triggers. This makes sense in light of the fact that *emotion* is defined as *e + motion*, which means to evoke *(e)* movement *(motion)*. So, an *emotion* triggers an inner movement or reaction becoming our third domain of inner movement. So now it must seem quite apparent that if we change the thoughts we attach to our feelings during an experience, our *emotional* triggers can be reprogrammed so we can perceive and react to the same experience *differently*. The next time the experience occurs, an "updated" emotion or pairing of feeling and thought triggers a *different* reaction. If the thought paired with the feeling remains the same, our next reaction to the experience simply becomes intensified.

So to recap, *feeling* is our first domain of inner movement. Then language develops becoming our second domain of inner movement as *thoughts*, and then *emotions* are formed from the "pairing" of the first two as our third domain of inner movement. Our *thoughts* can change how we perceive our *feelings* but *feelings always occur first*. If you don't agree, then remember, we had them *in utero* before birth. Thinking was learned after.

There are two other points I'd like to mention before I close this section. First, it is important to know that the switch from pairing a feeling with an experience and creating an instinct pre-verbally toward pairing a thought with a feeling and creating an emotion after developing language skills happens gradually *and* with overlap. As words are slowly learned some of them are paired with feelings to create emotions but when words aren't yet available or learned the feelings are still paired with the experience to create the pre-verbal instinct. Eventually, new words will be learned and applied and the instinct pairing recedes into the unconscious as a nondescript memory. But even there it still retains tremendous potency and relates to our vehicle of *intuition*…a subject for a much later discussion.

The second point is that this "pairing" process works across the board with developing both an internal *locus of control* and/or external *locus of control.* For those of you with some knowledge of psychology you may see a similarity to Carl Jung's work and the initial building blocks of the *Myers Briggs Compendium of Types* forming in the different stages and components of what I've described. Determining which mode or pairing with which an individual might feel the most comfortable operating may offer some insight as to which careers and callings are answered in our professional life choices and paths as delineated by the results of *Meyers Briggs* testing. And as we know, the careers and paths that catch our interest *and those we follow* are inherently related to and involved with our *motivation, Self-Trust* and *Confidence.* Learning to become comfortable and learning to utilize and balance all three inner domains of inner movement makes fulfilling our life's wishes clearer, easier and more well-rounded. After all, they do become part of who we are. It's just that our contemporary world puts so much *more* emphasis on our mental faculties and reason than what we feel or intuit.

So far, as a child from birth through approximately two years of age, we have felt and absorbed interactions with our parents and caretakers and now have a rough expectation or instinct for what we can expect from them in the form of nurturance and attention. We are also in the process of learning the communicable media of words for the mind by developing a vocabulary paired with our physical senses that labels colors, size, texture, temperature and sound. So far this has simply been pairing labels to observations and setting the stage for the first act of introducing the concept of value. Simultaneously, we also are beginning to perceive the distance or separation between us and those from whom we want attention. It is this distance and separation that will eventually allow us to apply the concept and recognition of value to ourselves and others.

In order to apply value to something, things must also exist that we *don't* want so we can make comparisons. Think about it. If you're aware of what you *do* like or want, you also must know what you *don't* like or want. Right? Unfortunately, in our culture we know more of what we *don't* want, talk mostly about that and, often, only have a foggy impression of what we *do* want. If you don't believe me, just make two lists: one listing the things you *don't* want and one listing the things you *do* want. I guarantee, the list of what you *don't* want will be, at the least, twice as long as what you *do* want. We even talk about what we *do* want in terms of what we *don't* want, or in double negatives. How can this be, you say? How many times have you said, "What I want is to not have to…" or "I wish I didn't have to…?" We also often focus on what we want from a perspective of what we don't have. For example, "I wish I had more time for myself…" or "I wish I had more money…" The inference is that it is assumed that you don't. It's crazy but that little word "no" that we first hear in beginning our vocabulary has *tremendous* bearing on how we approach life. Don't believe me? Count how many times we've heard the ordinary parent using the word "no" with a toddler and how many times the word "yes" is used. How else do I stop my toddler from hurting themselves you say? Without fuss or fanfare, simply redirect them. The less we use the word, the less power a negative inference will have in our child's life. The "terrible twos" will also be a lot less intense for us to deal with if we redirect more than using the word "no." Emphasis and repetition of any word creates an intensity and power in it. Other words with important meaning that we hear from baby are Mommy and Daddy. For adults it's love, sex and money. See my point? Why should "no" be any different? Not to belabor the point, but it is the word "no" which drives home the feeling of separation, rejection and the fact that at this age we may feel that we have little or no control over how the world treats us let alone how much choice we have in what we're allowed to do. Since it is one of the first words we learn, it has a long history of creating and recreating the feeling of a door slamming in our face. I have obviously digressed...but I think necessarily so. Now, let's return to our child and their indoctrination into our culture.

Introducing value happens extremely slowly over time. Remember, between two and, at the least, adolescence, we are still building a vocabulary to simply describe things and what we feel. Applying value is a dimension of mental activity which is much more subtle and involves immersion in a culture and family tradition in order to gain recognition and expression. It is one of the building blocks for giving meaning to our separation from the womb and our continuing to recognize the effects of that separation through our perceived distance from others. Let's explore where value comes from.

No matter what we need or want from others, the type of response we receive will trigger a feeling within us. The intensity we feel and the attention we give that feeling, and the circumstances that elicited it, are all factors that are dependent on whether it is satisfied or not. When we *do* receive what we need, want or asked for, we usually just take it in stride and move on to the next quest or requirement. But when we *don't* receive what we need, want or asked for, that need, want or request we initially approached others with is intensified. Why? Because not receiving what we need, want or requested *increases* our feeling of lack and yearning for it *beyond* what we started with and it then receives *more* of our attention. Remember, this process *is* dynamic, establishing our *locus of control*. With each additional denial or refusal the energy and feeling triggered by that denial grows and our future expectation of the likelihood of having our need, want or request satisfied diminishes.

In continuous denial, we can see that our feeling of distance and separation between where we are and where we want to be is getting wider. Through our growing *expectation* of denial, validated by our memory of our previous feelings, we become a "self-fulfilling prophesy" in repeating the *same experience over and over again*. As we become further and further separated from what we need and want and those who can provide it, the intensity and distance between us and others increases to the point where we begin to *see* and *feel* ourselves as **being** separate from the outside world. This is one of the first hallmarks of learning self-awareness, that is, we become aware of ourselves as *being* separate from the world. Meanwhile, as our vocabulary continues to develop, we accept labels of separation applied to us by our parents and caretakers, such as good, bad, tall, short, smart, stupid, etc. It is necessary to build a solid baseline of language before meaning will begin to make sense and even then it still will be a continuous process which will last well into and perhaps past adolescence. Initially we may not yet relate to or understand most of these labels, but as our vocabulary and comprehension increase we begin to paint a picture of ourselves from the memories of our past labeling. From this a perceived *"self"* begins to emerge, complete with labels assigned by the outside world. This picture is what psychologists call our *ego*. However, this *ego* is *not* to be confused with our social and contemporary meaning of excessive pride and contrived superiority. It is simply a mental structure yielding an awareness of a *"self."*

Our *ego* is a simple coalescing structure comprised of remembered labels applied by the external world, our feelings *about* those labels and the experiences that led to them. Soon, the memory of them will be fully absorbed and we will have been programmed to be triggered into "feeling" *emotionally* (feelings paired with thoughts) good, bad, tall, short, etc. when the labels are spoken by others. These labels and more will slowly become how we identify ourselves, especially in light of the fact that they resonate with the "who" that others perceive us as. Their first application and acceptance will occur within our primary family and close friends. As we grow older and make more contacts outside our family and circle of friends, our assigned labels may be perceived similarly but, more often than not, will shift to a meaning that's perceived *differently* from those in our family circle. After all, strangers don't know us as well as our family and friends. This will have the effect of broadening our perceived identity, theirs and ours, while creating difficulty, if not contrast, as to *how* or *why* we may be perceived differently by our family circle and those outside of it. As we perceive our differing identity qualities as applied by our family circle and outside contacts we may begin to prefer and acquiesce to some labels over others due to their ability to gain the attention and nurturance that we need or want from them. The ones that we no longer receive positive responses from will be either denied or remain unacknowledged, but will *still* be a retained memory as having been applied to us. Hence, we will still resonate with it but just not outwardly. This is one of the first conflicts in how we wish to present ourselves and will confuse the clarity we might have about who we are. This confusion will intensify the feeling of separation but will also cause us to look *at* our *"self"* and question why we might be perceived the way we are by some and not others. Depending on the age we are, the questioning may not be as much in verbal terms due to the continuing need for more depth in understanding language but perhaps sensed more as an "uncomfortable" feeling corresponding to a feeling we, as adults, might have as seeming to be incongruent or out of phase. In psychological terms we might call this *cognitive dissonance*. This is where our values and assumptions, desired or not, don't match our perceived reality.

The progression of developing and integrating these labels and qualities and forming a perspective of *self* that is composed of more than just feelings happens very slowly. It occurs much the same way as we might gather ingredients to prepare a meal, having multiple steps before the completion of the final dish. We could also say that the dish is more than the sum of its ingredients. That is, the structure for defining the *self* and the world is much more than just the composite of its labels and different relationships. This growing coalescence lends itself to a developing *self*-awareness much like a group of elements produce a compound that exhibits characteristics different, and more than what's exhibited by any one of them independently. Another way to describe it would be like differing weather factors coming together to create a perfect storm; something which surpasses the force or intensity of any one of its meteorological components.

Up to this point our child has probably progressed into school and through a couple of grades, putting them somewhere between five and eight years of age. We see that our notion of *value* has only started to build as the realization of our growing separation from others emerges through the applying of labels of character and the responses of others to us and their chosen labels for us. Because the mind works on the separation of experiences through labeling, and the more developed and "in control" our mental vehicle becomes, the more it makes sense that we feel an increasing sense of *being separate* from and definable by others. As that structure coalesces, our perceived *self* or *identity* begins to emerge, which psychologists call our *ego*. As the responses we receive from others begin to differ, the more our perception of our *self* begins to split and the more confusion we have about how to identify ourselves. It's this difference or *cognitive dissonance* that leads us into our next section on the *shadow*.

Shadow, Shame & Defense Mechanisms

We are at the point now where we, as the child have begun to see a differentiation or contrast in the responses we receive from our family circle, close friends and the outside world. This contrast is not only just between family, friends and the world but is even made up of different responses to the same labels. This in itself is enough to be confusing to a newly developing mind struggling to achieve a sense of consistency and continuity in how to comprehend and deal with the world. Remember, the animal part of us wants to make things easy and automatic. Contrasting experiences don't allow us to do that and keep us working toward perceiving a consistent familiarity.

This develops mental flexibility. Flexibility is one of the *"self's"* or *ego's* best tools for survival. This becomes evident later on.

Some of the responses we receive will be pleasing, in that they lead toward answering our needs and wants. Others won't be. Obviously, the behaviors that lead to the ones that do we'll utilize much more frequently. The ones that fall flat or are "off" will produce a dilemma. The dilemma will be that there is a disconnect between the *same* behaviors used to obtain the *same* objectives, but they receive *contrasting* responses from different people. In order for us to have a concept of *self* that is consistent and understandable, these "off" responses must be "put" somewhere in our memory of experiences. The fact they don't feel good is distressing and our natural response to things that are distressing is to simply push them away. This initial pushing away will be a denial. But that denial will not change the labels or responses that we receive from those others, and they will remain active in our frame of reference comprising our perception of *self* unless we can, somehow, deactivate their validity in being applied to us. The labels I refer to are those applied to us by others who call us smart, lazy, stupid, tubby, good, bad, disobedient and a whole host of other qualities that someone may see us as. As we receive these unpleasant responses from others, our natural inclination moves us toward seeing *them* as unpleasant or distressing and to label *them* with the unwanted quality they've applied to us. This way we can handle them being in our world but they no longer have a bearing on how we perceive ourselves. Since we, as children, are still almost totally dependent on the external world for labels and material that will help us define how we perceive our *self*, the contrasting label we received still has tremendous power and validity. What we accept about ourselves as "true" is and has been defined by the external world. This is so because as children we are still predominantly subject to an external *locus of control.* In this perspective the contrasting label which has been applied to us *must* be accepted as a part of us even if it is distressing. This part of us that we accept as "true" and *don't want* to accept about ourselves is called our *shadow.* The mechanism which we have instinctually used to apply the label to someone else is called *projection. Projection* is one of our most prominent and prolific *defense mechanisms* used to keep our perception of our *self* acceptable to us and the world so we can continue to receive what we need and want from others. What we need and want are not only the physical requirements of food, shelter and safety but also love and approval. Approval is what we, as children, would understand as getting pleasing responses to our behavior from others. This approval is how we discriminate which labels we *openly* accept about ourselves. The ones which we *don't* accept openly are sent to the *"projection mill"* for disposal. This feeling of being "unapproved of" we can call *shame. Shame* and *shadow* are both co-conspirators in that they have the same dampening effect on our *motivation, Self-Trust & Confidence.*

At this point it's important to establish some clarity about *shame* and the fact that there is a distinction between two different types. The first type is *healthy shame.* When we commit to an action that oversteps our abilities and the results do the same, we are embarrassed and we become aware of our limits. For example, if we commit to doing some physical task which might be beyond us, we'll fall short, recognize our misjudgment and set our intentions closer to our abilities for future endeavors. We might say that *healthy shame* is a mechanism that reminds us how to stay safe, physically and "egotistically." The embarrassment serves as an aid and reinforcement toward more conservative future intentions. Unhealthy shame, or *toxic shame,* as coined by John Bradshaw, primarily comes from repetitive and personally diminishing childhood experiences.

In childhood experiences that evoke *healthy shame,* we are reminded of our normal limits. They *do not* have long-term deteriorating effects. They simply remind us of reasonable limits to our human abilities. In childhood experiences that evoke *toxic shame,* there *are* long term deteriorating effects. The best example for the distinction between the two types of *shame* is where and how it is applied. In *healthy shame* we, as a child, are told that the **action** we do is considered bad or inappropriate. In this way we have no lasting effects from parental admonition except to understand where our limits lie and to be cautious in future endeavors. In *toxic shame* we are told that *we* are bad or inappropriate because of performing the action. This causes irreparable damage to our perception of our *self.* This application of *toxic shame* also has a resonance with the unwanted labels we receive from others that we discussed previously. A negative label applied by others and its acceptance by us is one of the most potent *assassins of motivation.* It essentially deflates our willingness to risk ourselves in the future, with the desire to not expose our believed inadequacy or *inferiority.* In other words, to ingest a belief that we are unworthy or inadequate will radically inhibit, if not eliminate, any willingness we have to risk ourselves when there is a possibility of failure. In short; it sabotages our *motivation.*

I have waited until this point to bring up the word *shame* because we, as a culture, seem to have an intense and irrational aversion to using the word when it is applied to ourselves. Thus far I have counted over sixty words that most of us choose to use in its place. When it *is* applied to us, we have the tendency to shut down completely and hear nothing else. This is probably just an *emotionally* protective reaction. To prevent you, the reader, from likewise shutting down on first mention of it, I've waited until now to use the term. Now that we have an understanding of where it comes from and how we process it, we can be more accepting of its application to us because we realize that it is not only us who feel its potent effects. Virtually every child who has a family has felt its effects.

In this day and age, we feel so powerless that anything that reminds us of that powerlessness (an assumed state of inadequacy) is either ignored, deflated, *projected* or transmuted to a more nebulous or benign word through our use of euphemisms. Fat becomes "heavy set," nasty becomes "impolite," stupid becomes "not the sharpest tack in the box," etc. The important point to be made here is that the *shadow* and *toxic shame* are sisters of the same self-deprecating feelings. Whether they are, in actuality, validated or not is not as important as the fact that we, as children, *believe* that we possess qualities that are considered by others to be unsavory, inappropriate, undesirable and *shame* inducing, and wish them not to be exposed for fear of losing the support and approval of those whom we love, need and have invested our time in. We tend to submerge these feelings where they then become incorporated into our *shadow*.

The mechanisms used to defend our *self* from the exposure of our accepted labels of inadequacy, as explained above, stay with us throughout adulthood. They just become more sophisticated in where they are applied and *compound* our feelings of diminishment every time they are activated and defended against. These then *feel* like a verification of inadequacy. *Everyone* has some degree of *shame* relegated to *shadow*, whether for acts completed or indoctrination throughout childhood. The fact remains that if we *believe* that we are inadequate or bad, to whatever degree, *we will act that way* and become a self-fulfilling prophesy through our subsequent actions. The *feeling* of *being* inadequate completely sabotages our *Self-Trust and Confidence* and in turn sabotages our ability to *motivate* ourselves into participating in challenging endeavors due to our fear of failure and the exposure of perceived inadequacy being translated into *toxic shame.*

The most difficult experiences to move past the effects of, when we are attempting to motivate ourselves, are the ones that occurred *pre-verbally* and still operate from the deepest part of our unconscious. They arise within us as non-descript and indescribable doubt as to our ability. They originated from the experiences we felt as neglect through not having our needs and wants addressed as "requested" from our parents and caretakers and became submerged when our mental and verbal skills started to dominate our growing rational landscape.

Our inability to maintain a momentum for keeping our *motivation* consistent and ongoing is a universal difficulty that almost everyone shares, regardless of race, culture or family factors. It is natural for parents and caretakers to become absorbed with maintaining a safe and healthy living at the expense of their children's best and most needed support. These dynamics are not intended for allowing us to utilize other *defense mechanisms* in blaming our parents for our perceived conditions. I have presented this progression of events and developments in an effort to show that even with the best of parental attentions and efforts we all still develop components of *shame, shadow* and diminished *motivation* in at least some facet(s) of our lives. The sections following this section are intended to show the dynamics and mechanisms in play, the methods of how they sabotage us and ways to move around them, like a stream moves over and around the stones in its path. We can't "un-experience" what we have experienced but we can redirect our energies to where they will render them to a harmless passage in our history.

There appears to be a lot of disagreement over what dreams are, where they come from and why we have so much difficulty in bringing them into waking consciousness. There is even more disagreement over their meaning and how they relate to our everyday lives. But their meanings go well beyond the scope of what I'd like to cover here so I will leave their attribution to therapists. That being said, let me set a couple of ideas in place before I lay out what I believe is actually occurring in our dream state, in our waking state and in between.

First, what we call dreams only occur when we are asleep and the mind is not functioning. That means that when we are dreaming there is no timeline and the changes that occur in the dream are solely a result of our awareness simply changing what we focus on, producing what appears to be instantaneous "movement" within the dream. Daydreams are different. Essentially, they are not dreams. They are fantasies that occur when we are awake, and are simply mentally created stories or circumstances based on our preferences, fears and the memory of past experiences. We remember them easily because they occur during our waking state within the mind's linear timeline.

Second, most dreams occur within the "space" we were in before we were born, that is, *in utero* and before. Their medium and "currency," if you will, are *feeling* and *intuition*. I say "most" because if we are experiencing a dream half in and half out of our waking state, the mind still exerts an effect on the dream, potentially giving it a partially tangible order. In that case it is, essentially, bridging pre- and post-birth. From the perspective of our evolving human consciousness it is probably the best kind of dream to have since, it allows us to create a balance between those two worlds of participation. But for clarity's sake, I will just say that dreams are the most similar to our pre-birth awareness.

Third, memory that lends itself easily to language is only possible within the linear order of time where the mind can use the distance between *past, present* and *future* in order to communicate and compare between *past, current* or *future* experiences. This means the linear mind functions *only when we are awake.*

Please note that I'm only using these ideas as extremes so we can have a clear understanding of what is viable and usable throughout our range of awareness between our dream state and waking state. There are an infinite host of points between the extremes where differing explanations might describe which dynamic (dream or waking) is the dominant field in play. Here I am simply laying a framework for comparison. As I move on I will first describe the dream state at its deepest point and then the waking state. Then I will attempt clarity in describing the nebulous field between.

The dream state operates within the pre-birth field of awareness, and is free of the three way polarity of *past, present* and *future* that allows a space for mental order. Its communicative medium is an agent called *intuition*. Its companion agent conveying intensity is *feeling*. Since there is no mental order, our awareness moves through the dream by focusing and refocusing our attentiveness. Our change of focus manifests almost as an instantaneous "movement" between scenarios in different settings. Our ability to differentiate between them is facilitated by the polarity of being aware of something, or not. To *intuit* or not is the same as to become aware or not. Something either is or isn't. There is no evidence of cause and effect. Once we move from one scenario to another, there is no memory or imprint of the alternate scenario. However, if one scenario has circumstances that lead into or connects with an alternate scenario, a *resonance* or common vibration is established and a "link" remains between them. We then are able to trace our awareness from scenario to scenario by virtue of the apparent links or resonances. There is no *before* or *after* so it is only the connectedness that remains available. When we move back toward the waking state, our mind attempts to put them in order. It's this attempted ordering that moves us closer to the waking state and enables us to "lose the thread" of the connected scenarios. The scenarios are connected through their *resonance,* like a spider web spreading out in many directions, with no beginning and no end. When we attempt to order them in a timeline the web collapses and we lose the *context* of the dream.

The *dream* is always in existence with no beginning and no end. (Sound familiar?) It is the focusing of our awareness that makes scenarios seem like they are separate experiences. When we are in dreams, they are all occurring at once. Remember, there is no time. In other words, in the dream field, if we can call it that, there is an environment, much like an ocean, that is totally connected in every direction and dimension. It is all *One* (Sound familiar?) This is comparable to our spider web. If we step on a "thread," the whole web shakes or vibrates in *resonance.* As we shift our awareness from one part of the web to another, it seems like a different location but it is a part of the same whole or the *One. It is the limits of our capacity for awareness that give each scenario its borders.* Think about this. This is a very important concept to comprehend in order to have an understanding of the dreamscape and its dynamics. It is *our mind* that brings our perceived separation between our experiences. The separation of scenarios is only in our *perception* of them. They, themselves, are the complete whole which we can only perceive parts within the limits of our personal awareness. Simply put, in the dream there are no lines, no separations, no differences, no borders, nothing to define or separate it into separate experiences. *Our waking state is our withdrawal or removal from that totality of perception.*

It is also worth noting that whatever state of mind we are in when we leave the waking state to move into sleep will be the same state of mind with which we will awaken, but with less bodily tension and resistance. So, if we were angry when falling asleep, we will awaken agitated but, perhaps, without the intensity with which we were consumed before we drifted off to sleep. If we were worrisome, we will return to a state of mind with concerns relative to what we were worrying about but, again, without the previous intensity. If we drifted off to sleep with thoughts of relaxation, peace, a focus on something enjoyable or with an appreciation of our situation, we will return with an easy and rested feeling. The point I'd like to make is that when we return to our waking state, we will find it with the same focus we left it with. An analogy might be moving away from a dock in a boat and later returning to find the same dock but, perhaps it rained during our absence and its a little bit cleaner though still the same structure. This says a lot about our need for *preprogramming* before we allow ourselves to drift off to sleep. Essentially, we can "set the mood" or *prepave* the environment we return to thereby allowing us to put ourselves in a space that is much more positive and constructive when we awaken. *Prepaving* is a trademarked concept originated by Esther and Jerry Hicks in teaching the *Law of Attraction* through information provided by the Abraham material. What they call the *Vortex* is essentially where we are during the dream state. I'll cover more on the Abraham material in *Tangent Subjects*.

Now, let's have a better look at our waking state. From the opposite perspective, it is the awakening of our mind each day that removes us from the perception that "everything is *One.*"

This enables us to focus on little pieces of our existence in order to develop an understanding of our place in it. It does so by dividing our experiences into *past, present* and *future*; the mind's three way polarity. When this three way polarity is activated upon awakening, we have the availability of *memory, recall* and the input from the *physical senses*, the mind's "companion agents."

A *memory* is, generally, where a physical experience, its attendant feeling at the time, and a thought were paired and committed to the *past* on the timeline. It can be preferred, unwanted, of no matter, or non sequitur (out of the blue). Every circumstance we have encountered throughout our lives has been imprinted on our consciousness. This is why hypnotherapy is so useful in revisiting the past. Whether the *memory* is *recalled* or not depends on many factors. *Recall* is what occurs when a *memory* is brought to our current awareness or current point of focus. A *recall* can occur voluntarily or not. (It should also be noted that, when consulting a dictionary, the words *recall* and *remember* are almost synonymous. I will use *recall* from here on.)

When a *memory* is recalled *involuntarily*, it is because our encountered experience has elicited a familiar *feeling* that we previously paired with a *thought* and committed to a point on our timeline. Remember, our *feelings* occur *involuntarily* so the repeated feeling "drags along with it" our previously paired thought or assessment. Whatever we had thought about our experience at its last encounter is brought back into our awareness. We will now, most likely, have the urge to repeat whatever action we previously decided upon or took, if we were to repeat the experience. Remember also, this is the dynamic of an *emotion*: an experience and a *feeling* paired with a *thought* or assessment. The timeline is a necessary component in the formation of *emotions*. In this instance it will *feel* like *we just have to do* whatever we did before. Remember, *emotions* evoke a response. Since it is a *reaction*, it feels like the experience is *happening to us* (exterior *locus of control*).

A *memory* is *voluntary* when our train of thought has brought us to the *thought* that we paired with a previous experience and a *feeling*. Depending on how much control we have over our *thoughts*, we may decide to intentionally re-experience the *feeling* by imagining ourselves back in the experience. If we are *proactive*, it feels like the experience is being regenerated by us (interior *locus of control*). If we have minimal control over our *thoughts*, we will most likely be *reactive* and the imagining of the experience will *involuntarily* trigger the rising of the previously attendant *feelings*. It will then again feel like the experience is *happening to us* (exterior *Locus of Control*).

It is important to realize that since the mind is only a tool and we don't have to put ourselves at its mercy, we can use the mind as a gatekeeper enabling us to revisit the experiences we have been through. This will allow us to reassess specific scenarios without the additional task of fielding *emotions* we'd rather not feel. When we begin to feel an unwanted *feeling*, we simply redirect our awareness to a scenario we had better *feelings* about or change our focus to more general parts of that scenario showing more favorable or beneficial qualities, thereby allowing different *feelings* to be elicited. The more general we can perceive a difficult experience, the more easily we can allow ourselves some relief through allowing a different *feeling* to be paired with the experience. This, in turn, will create a different *emotional* trigger for future encounters with similar experiences. The whole idea of reassessing is to allow ourselves some relief from stressful *feelings* paired with distasteful judgments, thereby disarming triggers that only perpetuate the undesirable reactions leading toward compounding those undesirable *feelings*. As we think, so we become.

THE FACES OF DISCOURAGEMENT

The Seven Deadly Assassins of Motivation

These seven dynamic types of personal interchange comprise the factors that surreptitiously work toward assassinating the implementation of our *motivation*. They are: *exhaustion, hopelessness, toxic shame, perfectionism, procrastination, altruism and reality.* They are all the result of post-verbal training. However, before we delineate these causes it would be prudent to review what we know in order to have a clear and simple understanding of what *motivation* is, especially, in a contemporary perspective.

What is it that gets you going? Is it a comment from someone else? A sense of awe? Curiosity? A feeling of responsibility? The specter of fun? Each of us has our own trigger(s) that serves to propel us into movement. This propelling, this triggering, this impetus toward an alternate place or state of being can be called our *motivation*. Simply put, *motivation* is stimulation toward becoming active through movement. Now, we can qualify whether this movement is internal or external. Externally it is, obviously, an observable physical action but inner movement is what gets our feelings and the mind into action, like when we have observed or heard something and we tell someone that they or their action "moves" us. Essentially, this can be considered an inner stirring or even a restless feeling. Simply put, something in us that was once inert or still is now catapulted into motion. Whether it is internal or external is not as important as the fact that it has changed our state of being or impelled us to "arrive" there.

There is an old saying that states "the road to hell is paved with good intentions." The implication here is that even if we feel moved to act in the direction of our chosen desires and whatever the rewards or consequences, there always seem to be factors that not only influence our desires but also work against this created impetus and often have the effect of slowing us down or even altogether extinguishing our blossoming efforts and intents. The question then becomes how much encouragement toward movement is enough to overcome the inertia of feeling that it's best to leave things as they are? After all, our natural animal instinct is to work toward a stasis or a quality of being at rest that will tend to conserve the most of our energy. For each person, the required intensity of stimulation needed for movement is different, but I will say that this is appears to be a factor of what and how much *external* influence we have experienced in our rearing as a child. There are childhood circumstances that are very encouraging toward independent movement and other circumstances that are not. Our culture and how it maintains order, socially and through the family, has a tremendous amount to do with how active we are allowed to be in the pursuit of our own personal interests.

The next step then, is to look at the spoken and subliminal (unspoken) messages that encourage or discourage our action and how they interact. At the core of this consensus and degree of permissiveness, most of us begin with the feeling of hope. Hope can be defined as an often irrationally held belief (a preferred thought or premise) that what we wish will take place regardless of the current circumstances and regardless of our immediately perceived and/or observable conditions. Our hope is interwoven with our trust in our ability to handle life's circumstances even in the face of factors that appear to deny our desires and efforts.

The survival of hope remains the strongest in early family environments that allow us to work through our own thoughts and feelings but, more importantly, have been allowed to decide upon and to hold beliefs that are a direct result of our *own* personal experiences, feelings and assessments even if those experiences might run contrary to the beliefs and experiences of those who mentor us. This "permissive" perspective is often only utilized by a parent or mentor who has arrived at a place of wisdom and understanding where their most solid and trustable sense of values has been gained by trusting *their* own inner urgings, personal experiences and feelings, not the urgings or coercive influences of those who have not found their own source for inner validation and harbor doubts about their own existence and worth. Simply put, if we have experienced encouragement in our own childhood, we will be able to enable it in our offspring. It takes tremendous courage, patience and acceptance for us, as a parent or mentor, to allow a child to decide for themselves in favor of participating in an experience, barring life threatening circumstances, which *we* know has produced difficult or hurtful experiences in *our own* personal history. The contemporary version of this permissive action, in the extreme, could be equated to what has been called "tough love." It takes a solid and remarkable person to recognize and implement it.

In today's social environment, individuals who have been raised with encouragement in trusting themselves are, very often and unfortunately, few and far between. More often than not we find souls who have been indoctrinated with beliefs and perspectives of parents and mentors who have not yet personally found that solid, dependable and trusted place within *themselves,* garnered through *their own* experiences in thinking, feeling and perceiving. Those raised in this fashion tend to be much more susceptible to external influences as a basis for making life and everyday decisions and tend to pass on to their offspring this trust in and taking direction more from the *external* world rather than their own *internal* world. Those raised with the encouragement of inner or *Self-Trust* have, so far, been able to maintain a feeling of hope, and appear to have a larger facility for leaning toward what has been termed by psychology as an *internal locus of control.* That is, allowing directional guidance to come from *inner* urgings rather than external rules and expectations. These children have begun life with faith in themselves and *Self-Trust* that they have what is required to handle life's circumstances honestly and openly. Those of us who have been raised *without* permission to self-validate through our own beliefs are, ostensibly, less stable and less *Self-Trusting* of our own abilities to handle life and what comes our way, accompanied by an often unconscious need to cloak our perceived inadequacies from the world and from those whom we take our cues and life direction. Factors that contribute to our feelings of self-doubt and inadequacy I call the *Assassins of Motivation.* They and our reactions to them are trained into our psyche by parents and mentors who have *not* had the benefit of childhood encouragement and who have learned to operate more from a feeling of *hopelessness,* whether conscious or not. Anything that tends to dampen our enthusiasm, curiosity and willingness to "risk" success *and* the exposure of our perceived or possible inadequacies falls into the category of an *Assassin of Motivation.* Every one of us has experienced some measure of this influence. Its effect depends on the intensity, frequency and amount of discouragement and external directing that we have received as a child. Let's take a deeper look at these factors.

Exhaustion is one of the easiest assassins to see the mechanism of. We have all gone to work and had days that really test our strength and resolve. At the end of these days we have come home totally spent. Looking at anything else needing to be taken care of, let alone feeling motivated to do something creative, makes us recoil with a feeling that all we'd like to do is sleep or "veg out." This in itself may not be a bad thing, in light of the fact that we may have put noticeable effort into doing something that we generally think is necessary and acceptable in the course of maintaining ourselves in today's accepted standard of survival and that the possibility exists that we can bring some tasks to completion. On the other hand, our loss of energy and willingness to continue "doing" after, perhaps, being emotionally assaulted by someone, whether through intention or simple insensitivity to our needs, or overwhelmed by the stupendous effort needed, edges on a more insidious kind of depletion through inducing the expectation that we will never be able to bring our tasks to completion. This type of exhaustion is much more intense because it often ties into our second assassin, *hopelessness.*

Hopelessness, or the feeling that what we wish to occur has no possibility of coming to pass, is learned through experience. It is learned through repeated criticism and invalidation of our efforts, actions, experiences and intentions by a person with whom we have placed our trust and respect, regardless whether that trust and respect is love based or coerced by fear. That person may also enable that *hopelessness* within us unintentionally through love and lack of awareness, but it is more often engendered through the creation of fear of unpleasant consequences. When this occurs in us as children, a lifelong attitude and perspective is created, validating underlying doubt as to our adequacy and fear of failure in handling life's normal issues and discouraging any action that might create personal empowerment that could potentially contradict that perceived inadequacy. The underlying fear is then masked with a feeling of *hopelessness.* This is often perceived socially as us being "shy" or continually seeing the "glass as half empty."

The *hopelessness* acquired through fear almost always morphs into a personal feeling of *shame. Shame* is probably the most virile and effective of *assassins*. It is where our own psyche takes over and compounds the "inadequacy" training we received as children. *Shame* in itself is not a bad feeling, as it makes us aware, sometimes painfully, of the normal limits we have has human beings. It lets us incorporate a rational understanding of danger and implements caution in our activities. But when that fear becomes irrational and is paired with a pervasive feeling of inadequacy, we no longer see our actions as bad, but we see *ourselves* as bad through the actions we perform. When a child is reprimanded as having performed an act that was bad, there is still room to develop *healthy shame,* as the act can be viewed separately from the child's character. But, when the child is reprimanded as *being* bad for the act they have performed, it creates irreparable damage and becomes **Toxic Shame** in our childhood view of our own character. This learned belief mitigates any possibility that we might have any personal creativity or adequacy and assassinates any *motivation* toward risking ourselves in any endeavors beyond our remembered *toxically shameful* childhood expectations.

Toxic shame escalates into another set of assassins, **Perfectionism** and **Procrastination**. How many times have we told ourselves we'll attempt or finish something "when we're ready?" The statement seems inert enough, right? But what are we *really* saying? "Right now I don't feel competent enough and I have doubts about my ability to succeed" and "If I'm still in process I can deflect criticism on the grounds that I'm not finished yet." Right? But where does that doubt come from? Somewhere in our psyche there is a feeling that we're not up to the task. Somewhere in our history we have been trained that our best efforts are inadequate. Again, as with *hopelessness*, this may have been trained into us intentionally, or not. Neither matters. The effect remains the same. We have, again, engineered an insurmountable hurdle to success. In perceiving the task this way we are using our "distance" from *perfection* and the "incompleteness" of *procrastination* as our reasons not to risk or finish. *Perfectionism* and *procrastination* mask our perceived inadequacy and fear of failure and lead to reinforcing our *toxic shame. Motivation* is dead again.

Altruism may be seen as a spinoff of *perfectionism*. Our *altruistic* visions can often have an "unreachable" feeling or an attendant expectation of being unattainable. For the person who embodies *Self-Trust and Confidence, altruism* is simply seen as a direction or goal to be worked *toward.* As this person, we recognize that these are performance goals set by the world and our social tradition. We are aware and accepting of the fact that we may never reach them and that it is no reflection on our character or adequacy if we don't. But for the person who is afflicted with self-doubt or *toxic shame* this is a red flag warning us not to tread there. In this light we are reluctant to invest ourselves for fear of failure or exposure of our perceived inadequacy. This also compounds into and includes a flavor of our prior assassin *hopelessness.*

Our last assassin is **Reality**. The word itself is not an assassin but becomes so in the context of accepting discouraging assessments from others. This only becomes a potential hazard when we open our decision making process to the opinions of others. To begin with, others don't know our heart or the impetus that has led to our being motivated toward our quest. Most of us view a goal in terms of our *own* perceived abilities. When we observe what others are doing we often tell them about the *reality* of things but we must remember that it is only from *our* perspective and that all *reality is subjective.* So the opinion we offer others is not commensurate with *their* personal goals but with our *own.* So when we *receive* an opinion based on values and perspectives other than our own, it will likely feel to us like a discouragement or criticism. And, generally, because the majority of us focus on why we *can't* do something, *not* why we *can*, it tends to become a crushing blow to our attempt to empower our *motivation*.

We are a social culture that has been becoming more and more invested in our external environment rather than what we know or feel inside. Feeling our heart is no longer a valid or acceptable reason for the choices we make in our day-to-day endeavors. At every turn we are now required to submit validation, justification, proof, documentation and various forms of tangible evidence for approval of our choices by the world around us. I believe this is a function of our growing breakneck pace, ballooning population, diminishing food production, dwindling personal space and heightening competition that our attention has been increasingly more drawn to who and what is outside of us rather than inside. It has caused most of us to become deaf and mute, relative to our true nature. In this light is it any wonder that the *Assassins of Motivation* have taken on such awesome power? This makes redeeming our *Self-Trust and Confidence* on all the more daunting task and vitally necessity for our spirit to survive. Yet, there is still a small portion of us who are aware of this and are working to recreate ways to access our inner power for *intuitive* growth and self-determination. The current social emotional blackmail that silences our *intuitive* urges and "knowing" in favor of social belonging and worldly support, which has been substituted for the loss of our family structure, cannot outlast our heart and its thirst to become aware and express love. Our *intuitive* self is at the root of our true identity. It existed first. We are not so far gone, it is still doable.

SELF-TRUST & MOTIVATION:
The Eternal Dance

From a Therapist's Perspective

THE URGE

The First Experience: Separation

In the womb we are safe, secure and comfortably encased in a warm and close environment. There is nothing we want or need and have no knowledge that there is anything different. This, for us, is essentially heaven, nirvana or paradise. Our consciousness is not fully invested in the physical body and our senses register as much as an adult would hear the mumbled whispers of distant voices. We float in a warm, peaceful limbo. When our birth occurs, a massive trauma reverberates through us. Our soft and warm dream is exchanged for a cold, dry, stark and noisy environment, but the most poignant effect would be the overwhelming sense of separation and disconnect from our mother and our symbiotic physical and emotional rapport with her. What compounds the feeling is that we have no understanding or awareness of *what* we're missing but that something is now causing us pain. Having been removed from operating totally within each other's emotional and physical space, this, essentially, becomes our first major loss. Having no way to conceive, think of, or process this separation, its effects dominate our entire awareness in an overwhelming fashion, much like a fish that has been thrown out of the water onto dry land. The only way to begin to comprehend the experience is referencing it against a vague memory of having been in water. This is our first experience with polarity, giving us the urge to replace what was lost. This vague, indescribable memory will lie behind every thought that will form within us. In order to perceive this experience as an adult, we would have to completely bypass the thinking process. For most individuals with the need to remain in control of our lives, this will be impossible. Yet, the urge will remain and have a subliminally powerful effect over every endeavor we will invest our time in.

Since we have no experience relating in any other mode than direct symbiosis, there has never been a language or a need to relate in any other way. The separation creates that need and the polarized environment it exists in. As our experience and growth deepen, it now becomes necessary for our awareness to expand. We must first realize that a change *has* taken place and then move past simply reacting to, let alone perceiving, that there is now a difference. That perceiving requires some form of memory in order to make the comparison. This is our first exposure to time and memory. There is nothing else to compare it to. Our mind now begins the arduous struggle with cognition. This imprint of separation is so powerful and so all-encompassing that there is no recognition of a difference. We are the fish having lived in the ocean suddenly being thrust on land. What could we possibly make of it? Imagine the irrational and indescribable longing it would create within us. This longing to return to our prior state is what powers our every urge toward attempting to compensate for or recreate our prior balance. That longing comes from an indescribable place where we, essentially, would not nor could not perceive it as rebalancing. There is no comprehension other than the pain of something missing. This must be accomplished through our mind and senses; all of which are time constricted and earthly bound and yet to be developed. Our birth has thrust us into a dimension that is so alien to us that all we feel is the urge to return to the bliss of oblivion with no comprehension as to where the urge came from or why we have it. Our first task is to recognize what has happened and our next is to learn to navigate the new waters. Both tasks require developing tools to interact with the new environment.

As our animal nature starts to surface and our reactions to it begin to form, a polarity develops between the urge to return to the oblivion of the womb and the physical urge to survive. This becomes a tug of war between what are traditionally known as *Thanatos* and *Eros.*

Thanatos is the Greek spirit of death often found with his brother *Hypnos*, the spirit of sleep. It should be noted that the death *Thanatos* brings is a peaceful one. It should not be confused with the urge toward recklessness, which would bring death of a violent nature as represented by the spirit *Keres*, the spirit of slaughter and disease. The urge toward death presents in many forms and has gone through many changes so that it remains a presence in our culture and our perception of the human condition. One of its permutations is as a label applied to Freud's "Death Instinct" by one of his followers, Wilhelm Stekel (1868-1940). It refers to a wish toward death, self-destruction and the wish to return to an inanimate or inorganic state. This permutation is an obvious representative of the urge toward oblivion. However, other perspectives we learn as adults are a bit more disguised and subtle, such as the behavioral attitudinal adjustments we incorporate to "get to heaven" as promised by Christianity, to reach "nirvana" as taught through the discipline of Hinduism, or to "be at one" with the universe as a goal proposed by those adhering to Zen or a metaphysically oriented way of life. These are just a few of the many socially taught disciplines and beliefs that have morphed our perspective while still focusing on attaining a diffused state of intangible being, namely, oblivion. In all these methods and more the urge to return may be subliminal but remains present in any case.

Eros is a different story. There are so many types of striving for survival that we can see evidence of its being in play in nearly every aspect of tangible life experience. However, there is a bit of confusion to clear up. *Eros,* in the Greek pantheon, was the god of love and his Roman counterpart was *Cupid.* Both were representatives of desire, which crystallizes the polarity of our separation from each other leading to our urge to eliminate that separation by reuniting through sex, much like the universe attempts to neutralize any other nature generated polarity. Freud's word for *Eros* was libido. With Freud, and through contemporary perspectives, libido is considered to be the *urge* to procreate and perpetuate our species. That reasoning is an embellishment and a bit more philosophical and purpose oriented than the simple urge toward pleasure and release from the bonds of the physical world through orgasm. This may seem a bit more confusing, as it *operates* as the urge toward orgasm which, essentially, briefly touches *Thanatos,* or oblivion, when it occurs. But it is the *separation* that is the domain of *Eros.* The urge toward survival through struggle and competition is often confused with the urge toward procreation. *Eros,* in its opposition to *Thanatos,* is the drive toward separation, dominance and distinction from the rest of our herd. It is, primarily, our growing animal urge to survive through control and domination over the environment in which it finds itself. Essentially, *Eros* strives to keep the polarity alive and even expand it, but *Thanatos* seeks to eliminate it. If we apply metaphysical terms, *Eros* corresponds with involution (dispersing and dividing) and *Thanatos* corresponds with evolution (collecting and uniting). If we stretch the point even further, we could compare *Eros* to matter and *Thanatos* to energy.

Whether conscious or not, these two drives are *always* active within us while we have a physical body. Our mind, which is *erotic* by nature, is the most comfortable when dealing with *Eros* and totally inept when dealing with *Thanatos*. *Eros* is time constricted. It operates within the framework of before, during and after. *Thanatos* is the timeless. Its framework is born of the timeless, peaceful, empty dimension of oblivion. It is this difference that causes us the most confusion when we attempt to reconcile our daily challenges, especially when we attempt to adhere to values born of judgments from a seemingly intangible and timeless nature such as our religions only imply. It should also be noted that the separation of the sexes that creates desire and attraction is regulated by the dimension of *Eros* but is powered by the dimension of *Thanatos*. Hence, we have both a drive to satisfy "lust" and an urge to create "unity." These two paradoxical urges, or *primal polarity,* power every action or inaction that we choose to take regardless of whether we are conscious of them or not...not usually being the case.

The Shift to a More Tangible Polarity

Since the time we were thrust into the physical environment, all of our attention has been absorbed by what we are feeling in terms of our separation from our previous warm, innocuous and peaceful existence. The urge to return to oblivion is most certainly still present but contending with our physical senses and needs is taking on a most overwhelming demand for our attention and efforts. As a result, the urge for *Thanatos* slowly and quietly recedes into the periphery of our awareness as our more present and immediate physical concerns take center stage.

The original separation from the womb has created a tremendous gulf between the dimensions of tangible and intangible, resulting in an unimaginable feeling of loss. Yet, the longer we remain in the physical world, the more we find ourselves primarily focusing on the tangible, if only due to its persistent and all-encompassing presence overwhelming our awareness of the intangible. To add to the influence of the physical, the awakening of our physical senses dramatically augments the dominance of the tangible and physical world, and the subtlety of the remembered peace and oblivion of *Thanatos* more easily slips beneath the threshold of our growing attention toward our physical world. Its powerful influence may slip, but its effects, whether we are conscious of them or not, remain a powerful nameless, indescribable urge beneath the threshold of our consciousness. The only difference is that it is no longer in the forefront of our attention. It has been "pushed below the water level." This physical world of *Eros* has been advancing on us like an army of shouting voices entering a room where only whispers were once heard before. The whispers of *Thanatos* have simply retreated below the threshold of attention through being dominated by the louder shouting voices of *Eros*. The subtlety of our prior and solely *intuitive* environment is now cloaked by the intensity and coarseness of the growing voices of the animal instinct of *Eros*. We are quickly becoming solidly invested in the physical world with all of its differing degrees of stimulation. Now, our attention goes toward our senses, elicited by our new polarized environment: warm or cold, light or dark, hungry or sated, loved or not. Our growing involvement in the physical world is now dominated by a process of dividing itself into preferences of varying degree as a new polarity is born in one pole of the primal one: the *mundane polarity* of pain and pleasure in the physical domain of *Eros*.

Our new concern in this growing environment is fast becoming the choice between what stimulation is more desirable over the other. It is this new separation, a *Secondary* or *Mundane Polarity that* promotes fertile ground for a capacity that has, thus far, remained dormant within us: thought.

What we become aware of always captures our attention and pain most certainly triggers that awareness. As we move through time, this awareness activates a growing knowledge of our preferences. This causes pain, this does not. This is pleasurable, this is not. The range of our polarity, especially at the age of an infant, is now resting squarely within one mode of cognition: the physical. Through this polarity, a timeline becomes fully active within us dominating our attention. The most important awareness within us is becoming focused on our attentiveness between "what was" and "what is." At this point the most important concept for us to understand is that *this tangible polarity operates exclusively while we're physically awake.* When we fall asleep, the voracious voices of our senses, the most dominant fodder for the activity of our mind, retreats and the softer voice of our intangible beginnings gently returns to us. While we're asleep, our *primal polarity*, or the polarity between the tangible and intangible, goes to sleep. While we're awake, the polarity of memory and preference maintains an almost irresistible grip over our attention. It must also be understood that there is not a point where this polarity changes like a switch, but is a fluid grey area where the influences of tangible and intangible mix and create confusion for the time constricted mind to make sense of. It is in this realm that dreams become available to the conscious waking mind. Whether we are able to make sense of the dreams or not primarily depend on how much of the *primal polarity* we have incorporated and balanced back into our lives as adults. But at this point, this concept is way ahead of our developing infant and a subject for future discussions.

It is this first or *Primal Polarity* between *Thanatos* and *Eros* that eventually earmarks our struggle to understand who we are. But now, at birth and shortly thereafter, it is the *second polarity* of the physical world of preferences, pain and pleasure, that becomes the earliest distraction away from the recognition of our essence and who we really are. Here, *Eros* becomes the dominating influence in our day to day living.

The process of *secondary polarizing* occurs whether we are aware of it or not, let alone the distinction as to which type of polarity is which, such as, hot or cold, or hungry or sated. The dynamics of time and separation begin working symbiotically as we slowly integrate ourselves with our physical world after birth. This is our mind's perceptual foundation and begins with what is commonly called a *tabular rasa* or clean slate. In other words, *the secondary polarity triggers the beginning of the mind's perceptual foundation.*

For almost all of us who are totally steeped in the workings and mechanisms of the mind, the state of perception that we started with from birth, or the *primary polarity*, has become totally alien to us. As an adult, our focus is almost totally involved in what has become history, or accessible to memory, and what is yet to come, almost always totally missing what is happening in the present moment. To us, the infant is an alien. Before we were born we lived and perceived in the world of the present moment with no comprehension of past or future. Everything that we think *about* ourselves is a function of what has come before and what we are yet to become or encounter. The key perspective to understand here is that our identity is what we think *about* ourselves and the experiences we *have*. To think *about* something there must be a separation from it. That is, there must be some distance between us and "it" for "it" to register with our mind and lend itself to being committed to memory or to become a projected intention for the future. These aspects are part of the time constrained or *mundane polarity*. Cognition is the process of developing the comprehension of, and the ability to, function within that timeline. The timeline is a function of the physical world and the medium that our senses use for conveyance. In the timeline framework, we can also see how the mind itself is actually a sense. Oddly enough, that would qualify our brain as a sense organ.

Again, for many of us, to see the mind and brain as a sense organ is a bit mind-boggling. (Please excuse the pun!) It's a stretch to think in this way only because many of us see ourselves *as* our mind. As an adult, when we have experiences outside of the mind's familiar tangible signposts, it can be extremely frightening and yet, at the same time, very familiar. When this occurs, we are reaching back into our *primary polarity* a.k.a. our *intuitive* faculties that we were totally immersed in before our birth. When this occurs, and if we don't "turn and run," we begin to move toward developing a balance by virtue of our movement toward a mediation between *Eros* and *Thanatos*. We have all noticed that when someone is dying over an extended period of time, they fantasized, hallucinate, they fade in and out, they dream, they speak from dementia and Alzheimer's, and exhibit all the qualities of losing touch with reality, or the
patterns they have developed for coping with the physical world that they had progressively built from birth. Leaving the body returns us to the state of timelessness we were in before we were born. What may seem strange is that an infant developing the capacity to become in touch with the physical world is acceptable and even satisfying, yet, to "lose touch" when we are dying and returning to the state we were in before

we are born is not, or is at the least, confusing. Our *fear* of dying is a component of *Eros* - our body's and ego's instinct toward survival that is aimed at preventing death at every turn. The *joy* of dying is a component of *Thanatos* - our unconscious desire for the peace and oblivion that comes with physical and emotional death and the release from struggle. Both energies are *always* at work within us. As adults, sometimes one is more dominant and sometimes the other, but both are *always* present.

So, upon our birth the journey toward developing the ability to cope with and function within the physical world, expanding on our involvement with *Eros*, begins. The speed with which we develop is dependent on two factors: our hereditary predispositions (nature) and the reinforcement (nurture) we receive from the physical world. Let's first look at our hereditary or nature factors.

Nature *and* Nurture

Our ability to interact with the world is straight forward and very much dependent on our *ability* to respond to it. If we are missing the anvils in our ears or they are impaired, we will not be able to hear or respond to sounds effectively. If we are missing any of the three types of the cones in our eyes, we will be unable to respond to the world relating to color effectively. If we have imbalances with our dopamine and serotonin levels, our memory and learning ability will be impaired. Our proficiency in responding to the world will only be as good as the vehicle used to process the responses. Cognitive learning may be affected by any number of physical or hereditary factors. Depending on the factors, learning may either be impaired or accelerated. The physical structures used for processing cognition will also be radically affected by the presence or absence of the appropriate nutrients required for physical development. These aspects can be physically perceived and measured. The process of nurturance is nowhere near as direct, thereby producing greater difficulty in its observable measurement.

The type of reinforcement (nurture) we receive determines our willingness to respond and to what we will be willing to respond to. When we cry as an infant and we quickly *receive* a response, we begin to learn through conditioning that attention can be received by projecting ourselves into the environment. If we *receive* attention, our awareness of and *our* response to being responded to develops a trust in projecting ourselves into the environment and our future *willingness* to do so is intensified. When, after crying, we *do not* receive attention, even after a number of attempts, we learn that projecting ourselves into the environment is of no consequence, especially relative to our need for attention, and the tendency to do so in the future is diminished, or in psychological terms, not reinforced. Sporadic reinforcement is almost as if there was no reinforcement at all. Whatever response we receive *consistently* is what trains our propensity and willingness toward taking action, or not, to acquire what we want or need. If we consistently receive no response, our attempts for attention will never be reinforced, hence, not take form. This is, essentially, our first choice involving the physical world: respond or not.

The fact as to whether we are responded to or not is only the tip of the iceberg. The *manner* in which we are responded to also plays a tremendous role in encouraging or discouraging our willingness to and *motivation* for extending our effort toward learning and developing social interaction. Most children grow to become discriminative in their responses, but infants will be much more receptive than adolescents or adults as there is, as of yet, no basis for comparison in their experience for them to mitigate and discriminate the variety in the world's responses to them. They exist in a world of *tabula rasa* or clean slate allowing the imprinting of almost any and every experience onto their new vehicle for memory, without a filter. Even as an infant, if we are responded to with love and acceptance as opposed to anger and resistance, we will be trained into expecting the world to respond to our interplay in a supportive fashion thereby encouraging us to continue projecting our needs into the world. If we receive an angry or resistive response, we will be most encouraged to refrain from projecting our needs into the world for fear of receiving discouraging, absent or even hurtful responses. As reinforcement formulates our expected responses in life it appears to be dependent on five factors for conditioning; *Encouragement, Discouragement* and *Apathy* as paired with *consistency* or *inconsistency*. If anger and resistance are the responses we've received as a child, how safe and inclined will we feel toward initiating interactions with others, especially if they remind us of the individuals who raised us and ignored, criticized or discouraged our expression? *How we cognize the responses we receive from the world has everything to do with whether we will risk voluntarily relating to the "outside" world again.*

This pivotal point translates into the whether we as children, will become *reactive* or voluntary (*pro-active*) in our expressions toward the outside world. We now have to ask, above and beyond conveying our needs, do we *require* a stimulus to *express* or does our *expression* simply come from our own volition or urge to express? That is, if we look at our developing pattern of responses independent of our needs acting as trigger, are we voluntarily expressing or do we have to be stimulated directly to express? Must we be stimulated into action or do our actions come unbidden and self-initiated? Are we *reacting* to a stimulus or are we simply *expressing*, unsolicited? This may seem like a very subtle difference but it plays a tremendous part in our individual attitude and how the expectation for our level of safety in relating to the world is conditioned. It will produce a very subtle blueprint as to whether we are *proactive* or *reactive* in temperament and personality. Do we trust the world to respond to us in an encouraging fashion or a hurtful fashion? If, as children, we can *feel* safe with the responses we come to expect from the world, we will develop trust and a propensity toward being *proactive* and *extraverted*. If we, as children, find the responses we receive from the world to be hurtful or discouraging, we will feel unsafe and develop a distrust of the world, with a propensity toward being *introverted* and *reactive*. In conjunction with feeling safe or not, our decision is one of the factors that will eventually and dramatically influence our feeling of competence in dealing with the world. Our self image will, eventually, grow into a powerful mirror reflecting that feeling of safety or not while leading toward growing individual competency or lack of it. This judgment will globally govern our approach to the world. In turn, our *ego*, feeling our level of vulnerability, will quickly take steps to insure that our circumstances and behavior will create feelings of safety.

As our mind slowly develops, we begin to acquire tools leading us toward being able to make choices concerning our perceived safety. However, it's important to note that in making these choices we will not always be conscious of making them. Many of us, as adults, are still *reactive* to the world rather than *proactive* and are unconscious of which we are. This resonates with the circumstance that the majority of people in our current western culture operate more under the dynamic of an exterior *locus of control* than internal, especially in light of the fact that we have become so materially oriented.

Additionally, it is extremely important to understand that as infants accumulating experiences and filling our mental and experiential *tabular rasa*, we begin to accumulate enough conflicting influences that color and condition our options for expression making it necessary for us to find values and methods for choosing how to act, not only between people, but between types of situations. This is fertile ground for the separative activities of the mind.

There are two fields of activity that our mind will concern itself with: first, the satisfying of our needs initiated by our separation from the womb and, second, a concurrent urge toward soliciting responses from others in an attempt to reconstruct the fast fading imprint of our prior totally symbiotic rapport (*Thanatos*) we had in the *in-utero* world we emerged from. Relating to the second field, the majority of people react to this *urge **below*** the threshold of awareness. Remember, it has been totally overshadowed by the volume and intensity of our having to contend with the physical world.

The mind has the potential to accommodate any participation in the physical world timeline. This timeline provides an environmental framework for the separation necessary to conduct our observation and assessment of worldly situations. The next challenge comes in first labeling, then producing a method for using the memory of what has been observed and, finally, struggling to convey the meaning of those observations as we grow into adults.

It is through these initial steps and separations, with all their interwoven feelings and the compounding of their interconnections, that the mind begins its journey. And to think, until birth the mind had only been a dormant passenger in our physical vehicle!

So Far…

Up to this point I've covered a lot of information and perspectives. To be clear, our understanding of the processes

I've covered thus far would be refined greatly if I were to distill the concepts I've spoken about already into a concise and definitive form so there will be no mistake about who or what I will be referring to when I use my chosen terms. In this light I would like to quickly recap what I've gone over thus far.

- *Thanatos* – is the urge to return to an undivided sense of oblivion where there are no needs separating us from our total symbiosis with our mother before birth, or perhaps even where we were before our conception. In it exists in the field of *intuition,* which is independent of time.
- *Eros* – is the urge and instinct for our body to continue and to survive amidst the chaos of conflicting tangible forces. *The mind* exists within the field of *Eros* and is time constrained.
- *Primary Polarity* – is the separation of a newborn's awareness between *Thanatos* and *Eros* upon birth.
- *Secondary or Mundane Polarity* – is the separation of our tangible world of *Eros* into opposing preferences geared toward our own continuity and survival. As it gains in dominance through increasing tangible worldly experiences, the awareness of *Thanatos* fades into our subconscious and eventually into our unconscious with its effects non-verbally surfacing only when early pre-verbal memories or traumatic experiences are triggered.
- *The Mind* – is the vehicle used for separation (choice) in the domain of *Eros*. The separation is enabled by taking static snapshots of experience and stringing them together forming a perceived timeline. The mind can *only* exist within this timeline. It needs the past, present and future to be able to separate preferences. It is most confounded by our *Intuition.* It is essentially a *dynamic*

force but uses *static* information to create its perceived identity through separation and comparison.

- *The Mind has two fields of activity*: First, it is geared toward satisfying the needs initiated by the separation from the womb (food, warmth, shelter, comfort) and, second, toward soliciting responses from others in an effort to recreate the symbiotic rapport (*Thanatos*) that was experienced in the womb (love, nurturance, safety). The first becomes conscious and the second eventually becomes unconscious. These fields, if further divided, are curiously reminiscent of Maslow's *Hierarchy of Needs*.
- The development of *Eros* is dependent on two domains; *Hereditary Predispositions* (nature) and *Reinforcement* (nurture).
- *Our Hereditary Predisposition* is the physical "equipment" we were born with, which will either support or detract from our prospects for survival.
- *Reinforcement* formulates a person's expected responses in life and appears to be dependent on five factors of conditioning: *Encouragement, Discouragement* and *Apathy* as paired with *consistency* or *inconsistency*.
- *Locus of Control* relates to a person's chosen belief as to which *locale* has dominance and control over our life circumstances: internal or external. If we believe that the *world* controls our circumstances, we are said to be operating under an external *locus of control*. If we believe that *we* control our own circumstances, we are said to be operating under an internal *locus of control*. Both are always in play and exist in varying ratios to each other depending on the types of experiences we encounter and our previous history of reinforcement with them.
- There is a strong correlation between *locus of control, introversion, extraversion,* childhood encouragement or

discouragement, parental apathy, and the consistency or inconsistency of reinforcement. They are related to each other much like in a matrix or a spider web, through interacting vectors of rising or falling influences. Their balance remains in constant change through acquiring new experiences.

THE MIND & ITS DYNAMICS

What Is It & What Does It Do?

As our interplay with the physical world becomes more involved, the vehicle for discriminating the *Secondary Polarities (mundane)* developing within us, our mind becomes more and more accustomed to separating and comparing the influences and experiences that we encounter. In infancy there is still evidence of the *Primary Polarity* at work. As we sleep more than we operate in a waking state, we still participate more within the world of *Thanatos* than in the world of *Eros*. As our waking state becomes more predominant, that balance shifts toward *Eros,* if only due to the immense amount of stimulation demanding our attention coming from the physical world. The growing need for us to participate in the physical world is aided by our growing ability to separate experiences with this vehicle as a result of our immersion. As the influences and effects of *Thanatos* are overshadowed by the dynamics of *Eros,* we begin to identify more and more with the vehicle we use to separate out our newly developing world. As *Thanatos* sinks deeper and deeper below the threshold of our awareness, is it any wonder that we begin to see ourselves as this vehicle, our mind? As adults, we have also grown to see ourselves as our vehicle, our mind. When we are driving, doesn't our car become an extension of who we are? Doesn't our sense of our expanded self extends to the outer dimensions of our vehicle? It's almost as if it has become the outer shell of our body. When driving, our car becomes second nature to us. It becomes part of us. Yet, when we get out of our car, that outer shell is left behind and our awareness of who we are shrinks back to the outer borders of our body. When we get out of our car, do we still think we are our car? No. The same happens to us as an infant when we go to sleep. We reconnect with that inner part…the driver.

To remember that *we are not our mind but that we have one* is the key to our personal power and comprises a major stumbling block in the field of psychology. To see ourselves as "being in the world but not of it" lets us see the tremendous power available to us in choosing to be procreative by *using* the mind as a tool rather than believing we *are* the mind and falling into polarizing ourselves through becoming solely *reactive*. This is the root of all confidence…*knowing* that we have the ability *and the right* to *choose* how we will participate in the world or, from another perspective, understanding that we are *allowed* to. The next big question then becomes, allowed to by whom? The answer is, those who trained us: our parents and caretakers. What we usually fail to recognize is that as we get older we tend to transfer their childhood authority to those who remind us of them. This leads us to all sorts of conflicts in developing *Self-Trust* and *Confidence*.

To understand the dynamics comprising the workings of the mind and its part in facilitating *motivation* we must look at the interplay of many factors: cognition, language, meaning, memory, nurturance, time, and much more. These domains are used by the mind but not always consciously. They interplay in a field that straddles our perception of what is both internal and external. Their discrimination and interplay is still determined by the consistency or inconsistency and the degree of the reinforcing of encouragement or discouragement that we received as a child. The mind is both a *proactive* and *reactive* tool and we must remember to recognize it as such. It is unfortunate, however, that in this day and age we *primarily use it from a reactive perspective* as we still assign our childhood parental authority to those who remind us of them.

To communicate anything we must first perceive *what* is to be communicated and formulate it into a scenario that is recognizable to others. In every experience, we position ourselves in a perspective that is aligned with our inclinations and the memory of our past experiences. This can roughly be defined as the process of cognition or, simply put, making "sense" of what has come to our attention; the "sense" being a comparison to our past understandings or mental constructs as a total aggregate of our experience. It is no accident that making sense is reflective of and dependent on our senses. This, included with our judgments, preferences and projections about the future, can be loosely referred to as our "*self.*" Each new experience and decision broadens its envelope of awareness of and influence on the external world, whether the influence is restrictive or catalyzing.

As our need to convey our experiences with others becomes our objective (in order to gain a reflection that we may assess ourselves and others *through* others), it becomes necessary to find a shared method of exchange, one through which both participants can, essentially, share the same experience. One of those methods is the spoken and written language. Others are art, music and mathematics, just to name a few. The biggest challenge lies in obtaining a true form of reflection, allowing and including unspoken nuances and variations in individual perspectives. The fact that we don't share all of our experiences speaks volumes to the difficulties in conveying any depth of meaning through our intended exchange. But, let's address first things first. Let's take a better look at cognition.

Cognitition comes from the 14th century Latin word *cognoscere* meaning "to know." However, our modern meaning for what we know will be colored by the contemporary flavors that the world uses in relaying or conveying the essence of meaning for what *we* know to others. This gives language a powerful affect over how we process what we come to know and how its meaning gets structured as our memory. The fact that the conventional definition of *cognition* also includes the word *re-cognition* is a validation of the assumption that the dynamics of *cognition* not only includes how we are to "know" what it is we experience but also how that knowing is structured in our memory so it will, subsequently, trigger the same meaning when it is experienced again. Simply put, the knowing occurs first and the memory, or our potential for *re-cognition* or remembering and then *conveying* that memory, is structured by the language developed by *each* mind.

The Transmission of Meaning & Memory

It's important to understand that our intended meaning for what we wish to express will *always* be tempered by the inflections and limitations of the language through which we must relate it. If the language has no word that conveys the meaning of anger, how would we then express it? This characteristic speaks volumes about the texts and scriptures translated from older languages that reflect an understanding and perspective of a style of living pertinent only to the culture originally expressing it. It may have added meanings or be missing concepts that our contemporary culture may be unaware of. This is the essence of the difficulty that we have in understanding the full meaning behind books like the Bible, the

Torah and the Koran. Their cultures, perspectives and styles of life express in ways that may be radically different from our modern day cultures and perspectives. Yet, their longevity lies in the fact that they possess some measure of the universal concepts that are at work in the contiguity of human understanding.

Let's take this a step even further. If there can be different intended meanings for words between different cultures, is it that far of a stretch to accept that two individuals coming from a history of different experiences, yet the *same* culture, would be faced with the same type of difficulty? The conclusion that we must draw from this understanding is that all truth and reality *must* be subjective.

The process of communication requires a *medium* to operate within before we can develop a competence in comprehending and expressing that essence of what we know or "cognize." That *medium* is the timeline. Its separation into past, present and future is just what is required in order to imprint a linear memory of our experiences in our mind. It must be learned, adapted to and navigated by us, beginning in our infancy, if we are ever to convey and relate the meaning of our experiences with others as an adult. The timeline lends itself to the cadence and rhythm of language.

As an infant, the responses we have received from the world have not yet been translated into the timeline with language. We are still living in a "soup of feeling" - hence, in the moment - so our ability to assess or judge based on a timeline is not yet formed. Because of this, the responses we received from our parents and caretakers as infants have no current or conscious *expression* in our adult mind and reside well beneath the threshold of our awareness. They only present as resultant "tendencies" or "urges" to express or not. The best we can do is to only acknowledge a nebulous fear or excitement in "putting ourselves out there." Even in therapy, it is unlikely that we will gain the ability to coherently express the pre-verbal experiences of our primary urges without perceiving the original experience in the linear form of the timeline, thereby lending itself to our language skills. And even if we are, to some extent, able, some of the intensity and depth becomes "lost in our translation." This difficulty is reflective of when we attempt to translate an intangible dream into the linear framework of our tangible world. We simply haven't the depth of language to adequately express the feel of the dream.

As we learn to perceive and navigate in the timeline, the transmission and translation of our feelings and experiences through a language necessitates the development of a useable memory. We do have memory of our experiences and feelings prior to the development of language, but not in a concrete form that can be, as yet, expressed. It is this "concreteness" that gives us the structure to discriminate and communicate our preferences. Memory and language develop synergistically. Both need the tangibility of the timeline to work effectively. As we become aware that *before, during* and *after* are relative to each other, our ability to express begins to shift into the timeline language of an adult. Memory then becomes a useful tool for us in the process of selecting preferences with the assistance of our *re-cognition* and *recall*. At this point, we are beginning to seem less alien to adults. Our perception is working more in the tangible timeline realm making it easier for adults and us to have a common, but very general, perception of each other's experiences.

To Express or Not To Express

As an infant our inclination and willingness to respond and express externally or not is established. It begins our dimension of how or if we will relate to others. It is populated, as reflected in the Myers-Briggs framework, with the dichotomies known as *introversion* and *extraversion*. The *Miriam-Webster Dictionary* describes *introversion* as "the state of or tendency toward being wholly or predominantly concerned with and interested in one's own mental life" and *extraversion* as "the act, state, or habit of being predominantly concerned with and obtaining gratification from what is outside the self." I assert that both these perspectives must, in their definition, also reflect the *urge* to respond and express or not; *introversion* including the *urge* or inclination *not* to respond or express and *extraversion* including the *urge* or inclination *to* respond or express. For the *introvert* this also translates *from* an *unwillingness* to express or respond. I realize that this distinction appears to be splitting hairs but I believe that receiving apathy, discouragement or hurtful responses from our parents or caretakers during our pre-verbal years plays a major role in whether we adopt a perspective of *introversion* or *extraversion*. As adults our *willingness* to project ourselves reflecting our needs, translates from our perceived *risk* in potentially receiving a less than desirable response from our parents or caretakers.

It is *before* the incorporation of language that the center of and inclination toward a focus, essentially the tendency toward inward focusing or outward focusing of our attention and energy, becomes established. This eventually translates into an adult's willingness to voluntarily initiate or participate in conversation or not. The threshold where one choice or the other takes dominance will be varied for each of us. The variation in which our approach and when we choose to incorporate it into our attitude will be dependent on a number of contingencies: *personal sensitivity*, the *frequency, duration* and *intensity* of the current external stimuli, the memory of past stimuli, the perceived safety of the present circumstances and, lastly, our *genetic predisposition*. As individuals, we know that there are some situations where we allow ourselves to be *extraverted,* and others to which we will be more sensitive where we will remain more *introverted,* reserved, observant and, perhaps, uncommunicative for fear of exposure to the dangers of our perceived insecurities. Let's look at these contingencies.

There are times when our *personal sensitivities* may vary. For example, when we've had a very rough day and we've expended a lot of energy into accomplishing the day's goals, or have simply just made it through a difficult day, our energy reserves will be low and we will have little tolerance for handling additional aggravations. Low energy reserves will tend to make us hyper-sensitive to outside influences that seem to be demanding our attention for their resolution. Methods of handling these experiences come in three variations: We can either "fold up" by virtue of feeling helpless and overwhelmed (*introverted reaction*), attack someone or something in the environment in an attempt to "drive away" the aggravating influences (*extraverted reaction*) or we can "feel the challenge" and become energized into pushing beyond our limits (*proactive expression?*). Our attitude toward *which type* of response we put forward is inextricably tied to the type of responses we've received, in infancy, to our projections into the environment aimed at answering our needs and forming our early conditioning, even if those projections only consist of crying or smiling. *Whether* and at what point we respond may also be determined by our current energy level. Let's look at one potential explanation.

For us *and* infants, sufficient sleep, "disconnect time" and nourishment will have allowed us enough time to rebuild our energy reserves after difficult situations and to have the strength to fend off disturbing outside influences. When this is so, our threshold, or buffer, for tolerating such influences is much higher and the point at which we will be triggered into reacting is diminished by requiring a much higher *frequency, duration* and *intensity* of stimulus if we are to be influenced. Conversely, if our energy reserves are low or we have become a low energy person, the point at which we will be triggered will be at a much *lower* threshold and we will be more easily and frequently influenced.

One of the contingencies I've included is the memory of past stimuli, which, I feel, at this age must be coupled with our perceived safety of our present circumstances. Previously, I've stated that we don't have the availability of a *conscious* memory but it should be noted that in infancy, when our language skills have not yet been developed sufficiently to render one, there are *still* experiences that we have that appear to be committed to a rudimentary form of memory that will appear to the outsider, and register with us, as an *instinct*. The animal or *Eros* side of our nature includes the *urge* toward survival. Somewhere between infancy and childhood that sense of safety must take on an additional face. We must then ask, "At what point does our reaction to the stimulus register as a change from only an *Eros instinct* to include a conscious choice supported by memory?" This point, I feel, will be different for each of us as we struggle to accumulate enough language to form the ability to *consciously* assess and choose between safe and unsafe situations and be *aware* that we *are* choosing. The separation that language affords us also feeds our ability to discriminate our "*self*" as separate from the world and in this discrimination it will be easier to see when the memory afforded by our learned language skills is being utilized.

Lastly, our *genetic predisposition* also plays an important part. Generally, when we think of genetics, we think only of things that relate to physical characteristics such as height, weight, eye color, susceptibility to certain kinds of illnesses, and mostly things that we can see physical evidence of in our family and its lineage. While this has long been accepted as being proven true through our own experience and the hearsay of our elders, we can also see indications of *emotional* dispositions that follow along the same lineage path. Even with this, with a little stretch of our believable limits, we can deem this as being acceptable and true. In this framework we can also accept the premise of nurturance as being a major contributing factor to growth and physical change. That is, we can believe that behaviors are directly learned through example and our reaction to those who have raised us. What might be a further stretch is that our *genetic blueprint can change* by virtue of changes in our diet, environment, and stress conditions bringing out attitudes, emotional *and* physical characteristics that may be foreign to our lineage. We as human beings are amazingly flexible animals. Yet, even as animals in nature, we are consistent in the expression of our lineage due to the fact that the only thing that changes might be our environment, which we evolve with and acculturate to at a *very* slow rate. We, as a species, assumedly being more than "just" animals, have the added flexibility that our human mind provides us. Yes, we *are* animals but we have an added dimension: a mind whose experiential processing enables us to hasten our propensity toward evolving and adapting to the changes we encounter in our environment. Let's look at some examples.

Learning vs. Genetic Disposition

As a species that has an evolving mind, adapting a general "civilized" consensus, especially in light of how we have grown to trust our senses and our external environment more than anything else, we have slowly become overly invested in physicality and what science has to say about every aspect of life as perceived by our senses. But in spite of the fact that our current day science is on the tangible polarity extreme of the tangible/intangible continuum, it brings focus and clarity to a struggle that has existed as long as man has been able to think. Namely, which domain originates how circumstance play out in our daily lives: matter or energy? That is; genetic factors or learned behaviors? The truth is, neither perspective can exist without the other and both have dominant and important roles in initiating and formulating the momentum of our existence.

Science has come a long way in determining which genes trigger the physical development and formation of what occurs in our organic world. Research into RNA and DNA has become extremely sophisticated and the tremendous social trust in what has been discovered has taken the spotlight, focusing on who or what we see as forming our universe. Through this research the scientific method has been reinforced as the dominant building block for the trust we hold in understanding our part in our world's existence. This has resulted in a plethora of information from mountains of studies done over decades looking for answers and validation as to why our existence is the way it is. What seems strange to me is that there have been, for many years, documented studies on the books linking learned behavior to genetic correspondents. The fact that this area of science has been intensely debated area may account for the fact that this kind of research has not been widely accepted, publicized or advertised, mainly due to the hard core scientific community's reluctance in validating and expanding upon research that it feels softens the cause and effect validation it so strictly adheres to. The suppression of these studies dates, believe it or not, all the way back to 1966. Let's first take a look at this seesaw effect as perceived through physical or tangible factors and then its relationship to intangible *and* behavioral factors. Our humanitarian culture, under pressure of excommunication from the scientific kingdom, has been monumentally coerced into focusing solely on the tangible reality of what has come to pass.

One such study by Rosenblatt, Farrow and Rhine (1966), extracted RNA from rats trained to perform specific behaviors, and injected it into untrained rats who, consequently, after being injected with the serum, exhibited the same behaviors as the trained rats. This showed that a *biological component could carry a trained behavior*. And of course, the hard core scientific community simply revels in revealing to the public any physical and provable basis that trained behavior *also* creates a biological component. (I'm being facetious) But the stunning, starkly apparent and replicable validation that their training has produced a physically viable component corresponding to a behavior, and that it can be manipulated to cause the same *behavior* in those untrained by simply administering what was initially produced by the first group tells us, undoubtedly, that we, as animals, have a profound effect on our physical genetics and heredity through the training of our behavior and attention. Simply put, we can change our body chemistry through learning adaptive behaviors *and* these may then be passed on to our offspring. Isn't this the basis of evolution? Why then is there such an assumed discrepancy between tangible circumstances that produce behavioral adjustments and intangible behaviors that produce physical adjustments? Wouldn't one have to assume that this rationale must be a two-way street?

Let's take this behavioral/chemical connection one step further. Consider a farmer. The stereotype that most of us have of a rural farmer is someone who is solid, patient, slow moving and "in touch" with nature, comfortable with her cycles of birth, growth, decay and death as being the natural way of things. Mind you, I am not speaking of the modern farmer with his business acumen, machinery and production line mind-set of handling his crops with marketing and financial implications in mind. He's a different animal all together. My focus is on the survival oriented farmer of our ancestral times who was devoid of all the modern innovations and contemporary business world involvement. This farmer may come from a long line of farmers with the same physical characteristics and attitudes assumed of those who have a strong connection to nature and the cyclic ways of earth, yielding a patient, deliberate and "going with the flow" lifestyle. His stress levels emanate from a completely different world of concerns than our contemporary one. Over millennia he slowly evolved this "man of nature" perspective and attitude. If we transplanted this man to a contemporary city setting, he would be tremendously stressed by learning and handling situations completely alien to his farming nature. He may either "fold up," by virtue of feeling helpless and overwhelmed (*behave as an introvert*), attack someone or something in the environment in an attempt to "drive away" the confusing and foreign influences (*behave as an extravert*), or he may reach into survival mode by "feeling the challenge" and becoming energized into pushing beyond his hereditary and learned limits.

In nature, evolution occurs with those who have taken the challenge and developed characteristics and abilities that allow them to survive within the changed environment. This might be seen as a variation of Darwin's "survival of the fittest." Granted, this may happen slowly over time, but occurs nevertheless. And remember, the farmer is still an animal, but has one assumed advantage over the animal world. He has a mind that can work with a projected future. In dealing with the changes, the farmer not only changes his attitudes and coping skills but, by doing so, literally changes his body chemistry to adapt to the changed food supply and environmental differences, and develops patterns of behavior that allow him to survive in this new and possibly foreign environment. Even though these physical adaptations may only slowly initiate chemical changes in his makeup, eventually they may be reflected in his genetic code and may be passed to his offspring. This is, essentially, the paradigm of evolution; physical adaptation contributing to a new genetic signature. Eventually, in the farmer's lineage, his offspring will arrive in the world with characteristics more adapted toward handling the environment than he was originally born with.

In the same way that this evolution occurs, we can see how a family may produce offspring who are radically different from their traditional *genetic disposition,* with the propensity for some genes to be either more dominant or more recessive.

The exploration of the mind-body connection is only in its infancy. Remember, the mind operates in the same timeline that enables the physical world to be sensed and dealt with in a linear fashion with the *other* five of our six senses. These senses are triggered through creating a *before* and *after* where their difference activates our perception of their separation in the physical world, thereby producing the field of change that enables us to be aware of being cognizant.

Unfortunately, in trying to get psychology accepted as a science, our categorizing of the human condition only serves to make our confusion and disagreement in dealing with it more painfully obvious. Organic nature responds more to the matrix of the prevailing energy variations rather than any seemingly arbitrary timetable. There are way too many variations in the intensity, the frequency and the duration of influences that a developing human can encounter as to classify the changes in terms of the "platform" direct cause and effect rests upon, which is accepted as the basis for all of the concrete or evidence based sciences. Perhaps, the advancement of quantum physics and its method of addressing nature in terms of relationship will allow us to become more appropriately equipped to define the structure of the human condition to the agreement of both science and the humanities. Unfortunately, the scientists of the world are still stuck in Descartes' mechanistic clock vision of the world. The more they try to draw the lines categorizing the differential flow by details and facts, the more complicated, convoluted and expanded their interpretation of the relationship between cause and effect becomes.

The fact that we still disagree on where to draw the line as to how we relate to each phase of our organic development shows us that there can be no hard and fast rules about what normal development might be. We can only observe when and how changes fall into place and then move on to determining the prevalent relationships and their most likely outcomes. The stock markets have already taught us this lesson but we still push on, looking for the "magic bullet" that will afford us predictability.

Each of us grows into a unique matrix of influences that perpetually rebalances itself as we encounter new experiences. The best we can do is to understand the major currents that we might have aligned ourselves with and then follow the flow to its conclusion or next juncture for change. The serum studies (Rosenblatt, Farrow and Rhine 1966) and those that followed have unbelievably scary implications for the potential of our pharmaceutical industry and what they might be able to do in manipulating our human attitudes and perspectives. A *"Brave New World"* may truly come to pass. With this in mind, let's move on, distinguish the prevalent currents and see if we can develop some sort of understanding of our mechanisms and *motivations* for relating.

THE METHOD

Now that we've taken a look at the combined variety of influences upon our ability to choose to respond to the stimuli involved in relating to others, we can see that the first determination to make is whether someone is willing to be more attentive to what's going on internally or externally? In other words, are we dealing with others as an *introvert* or *extravert*? Our orientation of attentiveness has everything to do with what methods we use to exchange information. As *introverts* we will employ a completely different set of communicative patterns and intentions than we will as an *extravert*. Depending on the extent, mild or extreme, to which we've been driven by our early experiences, the intensity and importance with which we hold on to our approach will vary. Both the *introvert* and the *extravert* are looking for specific responses, however how deeply the *introvert* pulls within or how far the *extravert* projects outward are generally proportional to how strongly our feelings of safety resonate with the people that we are dealing with. In contemporary terms we often call this resonance *chemistry*. But the usual application of the term is best known for its indication of sexual attraction. But that is only one dimension of possible polarities in which we've created a "charge" reflecting our position and perception related to each person or situation. Yet, it should be noted that we are affected the *most intensely* where our triggers for response are *the most distant* from the neutral point between the extreme poles of the characteristics that have been polarized or charged. Through that charged valence we will attract others who can oppose or reflect our chosen polarity, offering the opportunity to see and either neutralize or intensify the charge of our issues the most directly. In more antiquated terms, "birds of a feather flock together." It's not so much the attraction or repulsion that corresponds but the fact that we are "birds" dealing with the same issues. Those of us with aversions to each other are just as attracted to each other as those of us who give attention to what we believe we lack. This is the *Law of Attraction*. By applying our attention we naturally intensify our relationship, equally, with what we want as with what we avoid. This is a stupendously important concept to comprehend and address our actions and attentiveness to. It is a basic law of nature with which most of us are unaware and is almost solely responsible for us becoming self-fulfilling prophesies.

Describing either avenue in terms of *to approach* or *not to approach* still leaves us in the mind set of trying to "black and white" or polarize our lines of division so that we may more clearly recognize when one is more in play than the other. But here we must learn to be cautious. This puts us into a tendency of looking at the world in terms of macros; the pattern that science and the mind use in dealing with the recognition of either polarity. The mind is lazy. It wants to solidify the experience rather than expend the energy through staying open to perceiving the differences in the degree of ceaseless movement of energy between the poles. This is the law of conservation in action. True and accurate observation requires us to continually expend energy for the constant readjusting of our perspective to meet ongoing variations. In order to accommodate this conservation of energy, our mind, and science, accumulates static snapshots of the experience. This way they can make the *image* concrete, thereby conserving energy for future use in judgments. If we think back to the memories we have of the experiences that we have been through, we can plainly see that the *process* and *fluidity* of the experience is often lost through the *recording* or *concretizing* of it.

We remember in bits and pieces…the snapshots we've taken. Essentially, for the mind to create *memory* it strings together sequential snapshots of our experience much like a motion picture projector uses frames strung together to produce the illusion of movement. This is the essential quality of our mental timeline. It is our imagination that adds the movement we perceive in our memory.

Feelings, Thoughts & Emotions

The first domain of inner movement is feelings. They occur spontaneously and like a wave. They were with us *in utero*, are our primary domain of inner movement and occurred before our thoughts or physical senses. When feelings occur with an experience pre-verbally they are paired and stored as a rudimentary memory in the form of what might be considered an instinct. Subsequently, similar repeated experiences re-trigger the same feeling and intensify the previously formed instinctual memory. This memory also moves like a wave but is now stronger and involuntarily repeatable. As a pre-verbal child there is no capacity as yet to describe this new memory so it operates below the threshold of awareness. As we learn language the structure of the mind begins to form. As the structure coalesces, it begins to act *within itself* by creating thoughts - our second inner domain. As the new language expands *it* is now used instead of the non-verbal pairing and creates *new* memories overlaying the old. The major difference between the two pairings is that the memory created with the verbally developing mind also follows a linear timeline which is necessary for the mind to access and manipulate it, where the instinctual memory does not. This change makes the memory more easily accessible to our child's awareness since it now follows the timeline. The vocabulary that is attributed or paired with each feeling allows the potential for us to re-experience the feeling through repeating the thought and verbal trigger. This pairing of a feeling with a thought now becomes an *emotion*. *Emotions* are our own internally generated repetitive triggers. This makes sense in light of the fact that *emotion* is defined as *e +motion*, which means to evoke *(e)* movement *(motion)*. So an *emotion* triggers an inner movement and/or an external reaction, becoming our third domain of inner movement. Remember, *emotions* only occur *after* an event has been experienced, felt and then thought *about*. *Emotions* are the result of the mind's processing of the feelings and then committing them to memory as a static trigger for future use in events and thoughts.

So to recap, *feeling* is our first domain of inner movement. Then language develops forming our second domain of inner movement, *thoughts*. When thoughts and feelings are paired, they form the third domain of inner movement, emotions. Our *thoughts* can change how we perceive our *feelings* but *feelings always occur first*. If you don't agree, then remember, we had them in utero before birth.

Sense vs. Intuition

There is a *primary polarity* which is distinguished between the timeline (*Eros*) and timelessness (*Thanatos*). This polarity is populated by the senses and *intuition*. Thought can be paired with both, thereby forming an accessible memory. Since the timeline is the easiest to understand, and as it governs linear thought, let's begin with it.

When we see, hear, touch, smell or taste something, what happens? We discriminate a "texture" between the current experience and something we've experienced before and have committed to memory. It is the comparison of the *before* and *now* (in the moment) that produces a difference that catches our attention and registers recognition. This recognized difference between *before* and *now* gains our attention through the intensity, or perhaps "volume" of the difference between these two points on the timeline. The variation in the volume can be considered our threshold for awareness. The more intense the difference, the more likely it is to be recognized. The more subtle the difference, the less likely it will be to catch our attention.

We can reference a sense of intensity by comparing temperatures. For example, if we move from a hot tub at 104 degrees into a swimming pool at 65 degrees, the difference in the temperatures between the two will most certainly trigger within us an awareness of the difference. However, if we move from the pool at 65 degrees to a shower set at 72 degrees, the difference in the temperature between the two may not be of sufficient intensity or volume to trigger a noticing in our conscious awareness. Our recognition of the difference depends on our sensitivity level or the threshold where something will trigger our awareness.

It is also important to note that even though we may not notice a difference in texture, it still registers somewhere below our threshold of conscious awareness. An example of this might be that we are moving through an environment where the temperature might be below our comfort level but we're not aware of it. This may be so because we are preoccupied with other matters that are either triggered by a larger difference in texture or we may simply be preoccupied physically, acting or thinking through another issue. The point is that the texture or difference in temperature may not be intense enough to gain our attention. However, our unconscious mind has an interesting way of making its workings known. It has the ability to "put things in the path" of our moving attention in the same way we might arm a weapon before we actually use it. So, during our preoccupation with whatever might be holding our attention we may also notice the style or color of a coat that a passerby might be wearing. The meaning and usefulness of the coat are obvious. But because of our preoccupation we might not as yet make the connection to being cold. This effectively places the more subtle difference next in line for our attention once our action and focus on what we're preoccupied with gets played out and the intensity drops and is only then that we realize we are cold. Another example might be like being in a room where everyone is shouting and one person is whispering. We can't hear the whispering person. But when everyone else stops shouting, we can. An example of "putting things in our path" might be if the whispering person moved to stand in front of us. In other words, a more subtle stimulation may be perceived once the grosser ones are removed or the subtle one gains more intensity (moving).

It is also true that one or more of our senses may be more developed than others and have a lower threshold for being triggered. This can be exemplified by imagining that we have lost our sight or become blind. We now become much more dependent on our other senses. Our hearing and sense of smell become much more acute. Our tactile sense becomes much more refined. Our hearing begins to operate like radar listening for the reverberations in the room. The point is that each one of our senses is individually developed depending on our life experiences and according to the necessities for enhancing our safety and survival.

After our senses have been triggered our mind "pairs" with the experience offering an assessment or judgment *about* the feeling. This assessment or judgment, if sufficient enough in intensity, may be committed to memory and consciously remembered so our reaction may be prepared if the experience repeats. If the memory is intense enough and well-structured it may also be used to anticipate *future* experiences. Remembering our hot tub experience, we may, before stepping in, remember the previous experience with temperature and, if it was too hot, observe caution before entering. Remember, *future* is also part of the timeline and functions within the tangible framework of the mind.

Intuition is a horse of a different color and a lot harder for the layman to deal with. Since it does not follow the timeline, it is not subject to the same dynamics that regulate the mind. That makes it much more difficult for us to understand and put into a linear framework so we can exchange information about it. Although it can be rendered comprehensible through clever structuring of our language, it is still a very elusive and fleeting experience. Its dynamics work much more in line with the timelessness of *Thanatos*. A dream, and our inability to fully describe it, exemplifies the difficulty we face in attempting to bring it to the understanding of a linear driven world. Let me explain.

For most of us at best, remembering our dreams is a challenge. It is even more of a challenge to put them into a verbal form so they may be expressed to others. This difficulty in translation lies largely in the fact that our mental, and hence verbal, faculties follow a format that uses the timeline as its reference in order for us to express the dream's structure and have it understandable to others. Dreams do not do this even though we remember some parts in a linear form. Perhaps it would be best to first explain what happens when we sleep so we understand the landscape that dreams occur in.

Our mental faculties *only* operate in an awake, time constrained landscape. Not to belabor the point but remember that thinking *needs* the linearity of *past, present* and *future* in order to have a field or space within which to operate. This constitutes our waking state. This state is a temporal field for our mental life to operate within the same way that the opposing physical polarities hosting our senses (e.g. light vs. dark) offer a field for our physical state to operate within. The physical state can be exemplified by defining white by using the polarity of being opposed by black and vice versa. But there is a major difference between these two states of existence. Sense opposites such as white and black provide a state of opposing polarities that reflect the differences in our *sensing* of color, taste, touch, hearing, etc. *Past, present* and *future*, or our waking and mental state, provide a *three way* state of polarity allowing the *movement* of thoughts through time. Through these perspectives our *physical polarities* allow us the perception of *definition* and our *temporal polarities* allow us the perception of *movement*. When we "fall" asleep, our *movement* through the temporal world ceases. Time collapses. When *movement* through and the perception of time ceases, the mind is no longer active. It no longer has reference points for the separation it uses to operate. It can no longer function. The distance perceived between the reference points, *past, present* and *future* have melted back into the timelessness of *Thanatos*. The three way dimension has collapsed. It's like a house of cards collapsing into a flat pile. However, after we fall asleep, the two-way dimension allowing our senses to define our surroundings remains. The falling is, essentially, the collapsing of only the *three way* dimension. You might assume that the *two-way* polarity of the physical world gives function to the mind but it only provides the *field* for definition needed to comprehend separation. It is time, the three way polarity, which allows the *movement* of the mind, making it active by utilizing the separation. This explains why we can *comprehend the factors* in our dreams but not comprehend the *movement* and sequence without the framework of time. In our dreams change occurs *instantaneously* as our awareness in the dream is refocused. We don't perceive the *degree* of change, only the change itself.

When we fall asleep the body is no longer subject to the sequencing applied by the mind. The mental tension that was holding it in stress is now absent and the body may regenerate itself through returning to a state of "mindless" balance. The body has a natural ability to reestablish stasis when it is free of external factors. The mind is an external factor.

So, now the landscape is established. The influence of the mind has been "terminated" through the collapse of time. We are aware of the separation of things which allows us to *define* them but we are now in a sea of feeling where everything happens at once and everything is interconnected. This is the domain of *intuition*. Here, everything "occurs" in a flash, instantaneously with no beginning or end. It simply exists or it doesn't. There is no *before* or *after*. There is only *now*. What we perceive flashes in and out; exists then it doesn't...or never did. There is no past (memory). There is no future (intention). There is only "it is" or "it is not." When we change environments in our dream the refocusing of our awareness makes it occur instantaneously. Suddenly, we are just "there." Are you finally starting to comprehend the fleeting quality and evasiveness of feeling this way? Now, with this perceptual perspective in mind, we can comprehend the stress and confusion that an infant experiences, leaving that world of *Thanatos*, when being thrust into our polarity defined and time driven world of *Eros* through birth. No matter how we ease, cut, slice or dice it, birth *is* a traumatic experience. Now, consider this; dying is the *same change* only in the other direction...back into *Thanatos* or the dream state. It's where we came from. It's where we'll return to. Physical death may be a hurtful and traumatic experience before we leave the body but after we do, arriving back in *Thanatos* is orgasmic.

To describe our dreams or our experiences in *Thanatos, it* must be communicated with words. How do we describe a timeless experience with time constrained words? Words like perceive or recognize are inadequate in passing on what we feel. Perceive comes from the Latin *per* and *capere* or "to take" (*capere*) "through" (*per*). Recognize comes from *re* and *gnoscere* or "to know" (*gnoscere*) and "again" (*re*). Both imply the use of time as a reference point. But, time constrained words are all we have because our vehicle of communication, the mind, is structured with them. It's how we understand.

The "half in" and "half out" state we briefly reside in when moving from dreaming to thinking or from *Thanatos* to *Eros* is the alpha state and the only place where we can bridge the comprehension of a timeless dream to the understanding of time constrained and a mentally communicable representation. The difficulty is easily exemplified if we imagine communicating the interconnected dynamics of a spider web in the linear form of a tightrope. The best path for doing so is describing it in terms of what we *feel* rather than in terms of what we *see*. The better we can understand the *context* or *feel* of an experience, the better we are able to describe the interconnectedness of a dream. We can best communicate what we feel through using *context*. *Context* can best be defined simply by saying that we talk around a subject rather than in specifics to give our listener a *feel* for what is "in the center" of the conversation but impossible to be directly stated. The more depth we are able to learn and experience in our communication skills, the more able and proficient we will be in describing what we receive through *intuition* and what we experience in dream or *Thanatos* experiences.

There appears to be a lot of disagreement over what dreams are, where they come from and why we have so much difficulty in bringing them into waking consciousness. There is even more disagreement over their meaning and how they relate to our everyday lives. But their meanings go well beyond the scope of what I'd like to cover here so I will leave their attribution to therapists. That being said, let me set a couple of rules in place before I postulate what I believe is actually occurring in our dream state, in our waking state and in between.

First, what we call dreams only occurs when we are asleep and the mind is not functioning. That means that when we are dreaming there is no timeline and the changes that occur in the dream are solely a result of our awareness simply changing what we focus, on producing what appears to be instantaneous movement within the dream. Daydreams are different. Essentially, they are not dreams. They are fantasies that occur when we are awake and are simply mentally created stories or circumstances based on our preferences, fears and the memory of past experiences. They are easily remembered because they occur during our waking state, within the mind's linear temporality.

Second, most dreams occur within the reality of *Thanatos* and its medium and "currency" is *feeling* and *intuition.* I say most because if we are experiencing a dream half in and half out of our waking state, the mind still exerts an effect on the dream potentially giving it a partially tangible sequence. In that case it is bridging *Thanatos* and *Eros* in the alpha state. From the perspective of our evolving human consciousness it is probably the best kind of dream to have since it bridges the *primary polarity* and allows us to create a balance between our two worlds of participation, provided we can maintain our state of awareness in alpha. But for clarity's sake and for setting a standard to work with or positing the extremes in my explanation, I will just say that dreams lie within the realm of *Thanatos* and free of the timeline.

(The next section is repeated from the "Layman Section")

Third, memory that lends itself, easily, to language is only possible within the linearity of time, where the mind can utilize the distance between *past, present* and *future* in order to enable communication and comparison between *past, current* or *future* experiences. This means it only functions *when we are awake.*

Please note that I only posit these rules as extremes so we can have a clear understanding of what is viable and usable throughout our range of awareness between our dream state and waking state. There are an infinite host of points between the extremes where differing explanations might describe which dynamic (dream or waking) is the dominant field in play. Here I am simply laying a framework for comparison. As I move on I will first describe the dream state at its deepest point and then the waking state with which I think we've already been building a clear understanding. Then I will attempt clarity in describing the nebulous field between.

The dream state operates within the field of *Thanatos*, free of the three way polarity of *past, present* and *future* that allows for the timeline and without the tangibility of the mind utilized in its capacity for memory. Its communicative medium is an agent called *intuition*. Its companion agent conveying intensity is inner *feeling* (not to be confused with our senses or external feelings). Since there is no timeline our awareness moves through the field by focusing and refocusing our attentiveness. Change of focus manifests as what appears to be an instantaneous movement between constructs of different settings or scenarios. Our ability to differentiate between them is facilitated by the polarity of being aware of something or not.

To *intuit* or not is the same as to become aware or not. Something either is or isn't. There is no evidence of causality. Cause and effect are a function of time. Once we move from one scenario to another, there is no memory or imprint of the alternate scenario. However, if one scenario has circumstances that lead into or connects with an alternate scenario, a *resonance* is established and a link remains between them and we are able to trace our awareness from scenario to scenario by virtue of the apparent contextual feel and links. There is no *before* or *after* so it is only the connectedness that is apparent and available. When we move back toward the waking state, our mind attempts to sequence them. It's this sequencing that moves us closer to the waking state and enables us "lose the thread" of the connected scenarios. The scenarios are connected through their *resonance* like a spider web, with no beginning and no end. When we attempt to "linearize" them the web collapses and we lose the *context* of the dream.

The *dream* is always in existence with no beginning and no end (Sound familiar?). It is the focusing of our awareness that make scenarios seem like they are separate experiences. When we are in dreams, they are all occurring at once. Remember, there is no time. In other words, in the dream field, if we can call it that, there is an environment, much like an ocean, that is totally connected in every direction and dimension. It is all *One* (Sound familiar?) This is comparable to our spider web. If we step on a thread, the whole web shakes or vibrates in *resonance*. As we shift our awareness from one part of the web to another, it seems like a different location but it is a part of the same whole or the *One. It is the limits of our capacity for awareness that give each scenario its borders.* This is a very important concept to comprehend in order to have an understanding of the dreamscape and its dynamics. It is *our mind* that brings our perceived separation between our experiences. The separation of scenarios is only in our *perception* of them. They, themselves, are the complete whole which we can only perceive parts of within the limits of our personal awareness. Simply put, in the dream there are no lines, no separations, no differences, no borders, nothing to define or separate it into separate experiences. *Our waking state is our withdrawal or removal from that totality of perception.*

Now, let's have a better look at our waking state. From the opposite perspective, it is the implementation of our mind that removes us from the perception that "everything is *One*" (or the totality of existence perspective) and enables us to focus on little pieces of our existence in order to develop an understanding of our place in it. It does so by dividing our experiences into *past, present* and *future*; the mind's three-way polarity. This is the domain of *Eros*. When this three-way polarity is again active we have the availability of *memory, recall* and the input from the *physical senses*, the mind's companion agent.

A *memory* is generally where a physical experience, its attendant feeling at the time, and a thought were paired and committed to the *past* in the timeline. It can be preferred, unwanted, of no matter or non sequitur (out of the blue). Every circumstance we have encountered throughout our lives has been imprinted on our consciousness. This is why hypnotherapy is so useful in revisiting the past. Whether the *memory* is *recalled* or not depends on many factors. *Recall* is what occurs when a *memory* is brought to our current awareness or current point of focus. A *recall* can occur voluntarily or not. (It should also be noted that, when consulting a dictionary, the words *recall* and *remember* are almost synonymous. I will use *recall* from here on.)

When a *memory* is recalled *involuntarily*, it is because an encountered experience has elicited a familiar *feeling* that was previously paired with a *thought* and committed to a point on the timeline. Remember, *feelings* occur *involuntarily* so the repeated feeling "drags along with it" the previously paired thought or assessment. Whatever we had thought about the experience at the last encounter is brought back into our awareness. We will now, most likely, have the urge to repeat whatever action was previously decided or taken if the experience is to be repeated. Remember also, this is the dynamic of an *emotion*: an experience and a *feeling* paired with a *thought* or assessment. The timeline is a necessary component in the formation of *emotions*. In this instance it will *feel* like *we just have to do* whatever we did before. Remember, *emotions* evoke a response. Since it is a *reaction,* it feels like the experience is *happening to us (exterior locus of control).*

A *memory* is *voluntary* when our train of thought has brought us to the *thought* that was paired with a previous experience and a *feeling.* Depending on how much control we have over our *thoughts* we may decide to intentionally re-experience the *feeling* by imagining ourselves back in the experience. If we are *proactive*, it feels like the experience is being regenerated by us (interior *locus of control.* If we have minimal control over our *thoughts*, we will most likely be *reactive* and the imagining of the experience will *involuntarily* trigger the rising of the previously attendant *feelings.* It will then again feel like the experience is *happening to us (exterior locus of control).*

TANGENT SUBJECTS:
All Roads Lead to Rome

NEWTON'S LAWS OF MOTION

When we speak of *motivation*, it seems only reasonable that since *motivation* is a force that puts things (our mind) into motion, we should first consider the laws of motion, especially since the mind, the perceivable applicator of movement, is generally operative only through a linear relationship between time and space. This is not to say that it can't describe other relationships, such as relativity and quantum mechanics, but that the mechanism of its action lies squarely in that frame of reference. From that reference point we are availed of the use of memory which enables us to construct a working model we can look back upon.

In order to approach *motivation* from a scientific perspective (tangible and agreed upon origins), so there is no doubt as to the applicable parts, using Newton's laws of motion as a template would be highly beneficial.

For those of us who are of a scientific bent, who understand physics and who understand the depth to which Newton's laws have been framed and verified in ways that they might be applied for use in relativity and quantum mechanics, I will consider a human "consistency of perception" as our inertial frame of reference. This will seem like Greek to those of us who don't have a basic understanding of physics but will, at the least, give physicists a marker or reference point so they can allow themselves to move with my train of thought without shutting down before I get to applying these laws to the workings of the mind and how they are subject to *motivation*.

With that being said, there should be few impediments as to where I wish to establish an understanding.

Newton postulated three laws which have remained unchallenged for over two hundred years. They are simple and interactive and depend on each other to define physical motion in a tangible and observable fashion.

Law one describes the principle of *inertia*. Simply stated, it says that if something is at rest, it will stay at rest until something pushes it to move. Additionally, if something is in motion, it will stay in motion at its current speed and direction until something pushes it to *change* its speed or direction.

Let's look at an example. If a ball is sitting on the floor, barring any unevenness in the floor or an "errant" wind, the ball will tend not to move. If a ball is rolling, it will tend to keep rolling at its current speed and direction until it bumps into something or is stopped by someone. However, in reality, we know the ball will eventually come to a stop as a result of the friction created by its surface rubbing on the surface of the floor. So in theory, with no friction (an outside force or push), it will keep on rolling into eternity. When we look at how this law applies to motivation and the workings of the mind, we will see the "friction" as a force that the mind will produce which will affect our application of *motivation*. But for now, let's just work with our "friction free" example of the ball rolling on into eternity. The aspect of the *lack of change* in the ball's state is what I want to focus on and establish an understanding of as being called *inertia*.

Newton's second law says that if something is at rest or in motion, any push that is exerted upon that something will be equal to the amount of *change* that is observed. For example, if we gently push a person, they will move slightly in the direction that we push them. If we really shove a person, they might be thrown off balance in the direction we push them exhibiting a more radical *change* from their original standing position. If they were moving or riding a bicycle and we gently push them, we might see a waver in their direction and speed. But a more powerful shove would send them careening off in a direction different from their original path. How far off their *changed* speed and direction of travel will be will be equal to the force of the more powerful shove.

Newton's third law is what we popularly know as "for every action there is an equal and opposite reaction" or the amount that we push something will be equal to the amount that it "pushes back." For example, if we are standing between a person and a wall and we have one hand on their chest and the other on the wall, the amount of force that we use to push them away will be equal to the amount of force with which we push against the wall. We can look at it in another way. If we are helping a friend push an automobile that has run out of gas into a gas station, the amount of push that we exert on the trunk of the car with our hands and arms will be equal to the amount of push we generate through our legs and feet into the ground behind us.

So what I offer at this point for contemplation is the fact that since the mind needs the separative influence of time (past, present and future) for its workings to be useful to us, and then perceivable in a tangible or measurable fashion, that it can be also considered a function of the physical world since when we think we inhabit a space through that time continuum. From a temporal perspective, that continuum is linear. Anything that is linear in time has the *ability* to move through space. In this light the mind can be considered a sense organ that moves energy (attention) from one space to another. This, then, makes the mind eminently answerable to Newton's laws.

In the beginning of the 1980s an innovative perspective emerged in the psychological field that changed the way we dealt with many of our perceptual issues. David Bandler and John Grinder presented *NLP* or *Neuro-Linguistic Programming*, to the world. Shortly after NLP's arrival a young man named Tony Robbins took the ball and ran with it. Presently, Tony is probably the leading motivator in a world providing the most effective aspiration and encouragement toward personal accomplishment and dynamism. He is known as the self-improvement guru of the 21st century and with good reason. He capitalized and expanded tremendously on two essential *NLP* dynamics that were responsible for effectiveness in creating a laser focused perspective for growth oriented and ambitious individuals: *modeling* and *reframing*.

Modeling can be compared to **Step #2 Emulating a Successful Character** in the *Small & Easy Steps* section. In doing so, we can feel what it would be like to be successful in the field of our choosing. Step #2 utilizes *empathy* which is a powerful, innate dynamic that can, literally, put us in the feeling place of another person so we might totally comprehend what their movement and space feels like. We can then recall the feelings within ourselves when we are in situations that correspond to where we desire to be more successful and in control. If we adjust our awareness slightly we can also feel what it is like to be on the (+) end of the emotional scale and ingest the feel of an internal *locus of control*.

Reframing can be compared to using **Step #6 Using I-Dialogue**. *Reframing* occurs when we change the *context* of a circumstance so it can be viewed and felt from a different perspective, implying different consequences. We do this when we use **I-Dialogue** and include ourselves in their perceived field of accountability. When we and they both feel and accept a combined responsibility for an event, the shared responsibility shifts the need for the other to be defensive about perceived inadequacies and see the shared responsibility as a combined effort removing the urgency for individual self-defensiveness. The *context* or the meaning of the event takes on a different flavor for the other person and they can relax more into a lesser demand for performance and risk of exposure. This, in turn, allows for an easier and less threatening road toward building *Self-Trust* and *Confidence*.

There are many other tricks and tools that can be used to enable the feel of power and control in *NLP* as there are in *Energizing Self-Trust*. The name of the game is to allow ourselves to temporarily feel differently in a situation while we use the opportunity to replace the pairing of our previous assessment and judgment about ourselves through repeating the experience with a new perspective that allows us to feel our own power and control, consequently changing our older self-assessment and judgment for the new one.

In just looking at these two steps we can see that *NLP* is, obviously, another viable path for reclaiming our power. In reading the materials you will find many other resonant perspectives.

THE LAW OF ATTRACTION

The belief that our lives are determined by external circumstances is not a new concept. It resonates the most closely with the scientific method and scientific principles, as does the belief that our individual internal faith determines how worldly circumstances will follow. Our perspectives on self-determinism move cyclically within the polarized relationship between external and internal *loci of control*. This can change moment to moment or over eons. Due to the fact that all things earthly run in cycles, like the seasons, like the movement from day to night and back again, and the ebbing and flowing of the tides, the thinking and beliefs of generations and epochs run the same alternating course. Where a noticeable change takes place is where one perspective becomes so dominant or extreme that an awareness of the need to change our direction of movement between the poles becomes an overwhelming drive. In the early 1500s we felt overly oppressed by the dictates of religious dogma. The result: the advent of the Age of Reason. In the mid-1700s the Western world felt overly oppressed by political forces. The result: the American Revolution and reflective struggles all throughout Europe. And now, having begun in the mid-1900s, with the feeling of oppression felt as a result of our overly dominant scientific and technical currents determining our survival we're feeling a resurgent need to rebalance the scales of our beliefs toward a stronger self-determinism. This can be seen in our current culture's increasing obsession with personal and self-improvement, or the good of the many becoming more focused toward the good of the one, reflecting the need to come more "back to center" in our beliefs about what and who determines our fate. Within that wave of rebalancing has been the underlying force of what we have come to know as the *Law of Attraction*.

The Secret has become the rage of the 2000s. Its emphasis on our taking personal control over our life circumstances has energized millions into adapting an alternative focus to the "science determines the world" view that has been so dominant and so influential in overemphasizing our Cartesian view of the world that sees each person as simply the workings of a much larger mechanical clock, namely, the view that "what is" describes who we are and where we are going. The obvious absence of personal input has created an almost overwhelming and mostly unconscious revolution in our beliefs about whom and what determines the direction of our worldly concerns. "I think, therefore I am" has been slowly morphing into "I am, therefore I feel," giving paramount emphasis to individual self-determinism.

The *Law of Attraction* view asserts that we become a "self-fulfilling prophesy" when we run our lives on what we currently observe and what has come before. The premise is that "what is" is the materialization of our expectations and, therefore, a self-fulfilling prophesy. The contention is very much akin to the perspective offered by our greatest prophets: Jesus, Buddha, Mohammed, Krishna and countless others who assert that our faith, or our worldly expectations, determines how the world will manifest and unfold. This resonates very strongly with the belief that our *Self-Trust & Confidence* exert a major influence in how the world answers our desires and wishes. We all know how strongly these factors play on our worldly experiences, especially when we feel a lack of their influence.

Although some of the principles of the *Law of Attraction* may appear to disagree with some of the forming perspectives that I have outlined in this book, be assured that as the smoke clears and the syntax of what is being discussed becomes more crystalized and focused in both areas, we will begin to see a strong resonant perspective underlying the principles of how our life views and our perspectives on self-determinism are being radically affected in a similar fashion.

The last thing I'd like to mention about the *Law of Attraction* is that within its workings, and this is true of any changing methods and perspectives, there are, seemingly, conflicting viewpoints as to the objectives and workings of the laws. Those who initially meet the concepts see a method for accumulation as being its primary objective. But on closer analysis and by integrating the principles, feelings of a much deeper and more pervasive understanding begin to create a clarity about the workings of our lives and the principles of manifestation. I heartily recommend working with the Abraham-Hicks materials, as I feel they hold a resonant perspective with the materials and methods I have included in my modest book.

TRANSACTIONAL ANALYSIS

In the mid to late 60s a conceptual self-improvement wave washed over the psychological community involving Transactional Analysis (TA). Coupled with the encounter group phenomenon such as *EST* and *Lifespring* the focus on self-actualization and personal performance orientation took center stage. With their arrival it became fashionable to be seeing an analyst and the public became obsessed with becoming emotionally balanced amidst the growing stresses and challenges of survival and expected social conformity. All of this occurred on the heels of a booming postwar industrialization and a slow social homogenizing of the average American. TA became a preferable way to shake out all the cobwebs and project individuality.

Simply put, TA approached therapy through dealing with our ingrained childhood patterns of learning, fulfilling and playing specific roles in our relationships. The premise was that our projected image and ingrained behavior attract a complimentary energy that "fills in the gaps" that are required for us to maintain a balance in our relationships, whether that balance is healthy or not. Problems arose as it was recognized that the emotional and behavioral patterns originating in and appropriate for childhood carried over into adult relationships creating an interpersonal rapport inhibiting the maturing of productive and healthy relationship objectives.

TA's power rested in the fact that it allowed therapists to recognized our "defective" role-plays and their tendency to halt, and in some cases retard, our emotional development and alignment on our journey toward emotional health. The structure of the therapy suggests, generally, that in this role-play we may inhabit one of three perspectives in our personal relationships: that of a child, that of a parent, or that of an adult. The adult role was considered to be healthy and balanced and assumed a posture of making and taking reasonable and independent decisions and actions while being accountable and responsible for those decisions, actions and consequences The child's role and parental role operated together much like a lock and a key. The person occupying the child role would assume no responsibility and would behave as a child would under the supervision and stewardship of the person assuming the parental role. The parent, in turn, would assume all the control, responsibility and accountability for the "child" and their actions or lack of same. Both could then continue the roles they learned in childhood effectively eliminating the need to mature and become reasonable, accountable and responsible adults beyond their childhood emotional patterning. This effectively reflects the most intense side of an external *locus of control,* yielding the control of our lives over to an external entity; the parent held by the responsibility for the child and the child unable to act without the permission or guidance of the parent. Both were immune to the advantages of or exposure to having *Self-Trust* or *Confidence* which are necessary for the feeling of wholeness and emotionally maturity an adult enjoys in determining their own course in life. Both lives are completely dependent on an authority outside of themselves.

The roles of child vs. parent are very similar to the interwoven perspectives that are experienced in a family where a scapegoat endures the brunt of criticisms thereby shielding other members of the family from facing their own perceived personal inadequacies. Through performing a scripted role, the scapegoat, insures the family's continued dysfunctionality and diminished risk of exposure. The range of circumstances cloaked or shielded can extend from simple insecurities to blatant emotional and physical abuse.

In Transactional Analysis the role of "adult" is representative of the individual who has matured past the parent/child relationship and has taken their place in society as a responsible, competent and accountable person possessing strong *Self-Trust* and *Confidence* in their ability to handle the adult world and the myriad unexpected events that we all occasionally face.

The concept behind Transactional Analysis is a good one but tremendously simplistic in its assessment and addressing of relationship interplay. As *some* therapists have moved past their preoccupation with "behavioral adjustment" and more into changing the root causes of the "defective" beliefs originated in dysfunctional childhood programming, our road to empowering individuals with *Self-Trust* and *Confidence* is creating more peace oriented and effective leaders and individuals possessing courage, fortitude, vision and insight.

PROLOGUE

In some cases *Energizing Self-Trust* can seem to be a daunting task. But we have to remember that it's taken *us* a lifetime to arrive at the perspective that *we* are living in and, along with our learned behavior, we have also trained others how to deal with us and what *they* can expect from us in terms of *their* needs and expectations…even if those expectation might be irrational and dysfunctional. We all operate within a practiced comfort zone and it might take a short time to change *our* behavior but, perhaps, a *very* long time to teach others to treat us differently. In some cases, our attempts to train others to treat us differently will be like us pushing the stone in the myth of Sisyphus, constantly rolling back to its original position of comfort, symbolic of their deeply and fearfully resisting the change. In these cases we must assess whether it is in our best interest to limit our exposure, if not eliminate our contact with them in light of the fact that their influences on us will remain toxic to our *Self-Trust* and *Confidence*…at least until we are solid in our new emotional perspective. In other cases, we will be successful in enabling different and healthier relationships with those who before had had a negative and diminishing influence on us. In expanding ourselves we may even assist *them* in changing their expectations of rapport with others, thereby, assisting *them* in finding a place in life more akin to the (+) side of the emotional scale in their locus of control. Either way, it's a win/win situation for us to reclaim our *Self-Trust & Confidence*.

GLOSSARY

of Supporting Definitions

A Note on the definitions presented: These definitions are not meant to correspond to the definitions found in most conventional dictionaries, psychology text books, philosophy text books or any other media intended to standardize meanings with and for our contemporary understandings. Although in some cases similarities may exist, the meanings I present here are intended to show some word origins and my own personal understandings as to how they relate to the material I have presented. They are a blending of many different sources, including an *Etymology Dictionary* and *www.Etymonline.com*, geared toward allowing our meanings to ostensibly "be on the same page" when delineating the concepts I wish to share.

Algernon Dilemma – was originally an ethical dilemma presented in the movie *Flowers for Algernon* posing the question, "Do I have the right to change this person's personality and awareness even though they may appear better to me due to my efforts?" I couple this, taking that dilemma to another level with the statement, "The more aware I become, the less people there are for me to relate to."

Attention, attend – comes from the old French *atendre* meaning "to expect or to wait for" and the Latin *attendere* meaning "to give heed to" or *ad* (to) + *tendere* (stretch).

Cognitive Dissonance – is a term coined by the psychologist Leon Festinger meaning holding of two beliefs simultaneously that are contradictory to each other. An example would be a stated desire to not want to smoke while buying a pack of cigarettes.

Cognizance – from 14th century *conysance* meaning "knowledge" and later from modern French *conoiste* meaning "to know or be acquainted with" and from the Latin *cognoscere* meaning "to get to know or recognize" (know again).

Context, contextual – from the 15th century Latin *contextus* meaning a "joining together" or from *com* (together) + *texere* (to weave, to make). It can be defined simply as saying that we talk "around" a subject rather than in specifics so that we may give our listener a *feel* for what is "in the center" of conversation but is, usually, not possible to be directly stated.

Desire – comes from the 13th century old French *desir* meaning "a sense of lust" or desirer meaning to wish for, long for" and from Latin *desiderare* meaning to "long for, wish for, demand, expect." Desire can be used as a verb or a noun.

Dynamic(s) – comes from the 1827 French *dynamique* meaning "a force that produces motion" as opposed to being "static or at rest" and from the Greek, 1691 as, *dynamikos* meaning "to be able, force, drive, have power and be strong enough." It can be used as an adjective and a noun.

Emotion – a dynamic which is the product of the "pairing" of a feeling, experience and judgment (thought) that is committed to memory and has the potential to be triggered by future events or can be triggered voluntarily through the stimulus of thoughts. Emotions can be reprogrammed through an act of will through thought selection.

Eros – is the urge and instinct for our body to continue and to survive amidst the chaos of conflicting tangible forces. *The Mind* exists within the field of *Eros* and is time constrained.

Extravert, extraversion – The *Miriam-Webster Dictionary* describes extraversion as "the act, state, or habit of being predominantly concerned with and obtaining gratification from what is outside the self. I assert that this perspective must, in its definition, also reflect the urge to respond and express or not;

extraversion being the willingness, urge or inclination *to* respond or express.

Feel, feeling (not related to five our senses) - A movement of energy within us that arises involuntarily and elicits a "flavor" commensurate with its trigger and evoking an approach or avoidance involving an experience.

Hereditary Predisposition - is the physical or genetically generated "equipment" we were born with that will either support or detract from our prospects for survival.

Introvert, introversion – The *Miriam-Webster Dictionary* describes introversion as "the state of or tendency toward being wholly or predominantly concerned with and interested in one's own mental life." I assert that this perspective must, in its definition, also reflect the urge to respond and express or not; with introversion being the urge or inclination *not* to respond or express.

Locus of Control (LOC) - relates to a person's chosen belief as to which *locale* has dominance and control over our life circumstances: internal or external. If we believe that the *world* controls our circumstances, we are said to be operating under an external *locus of control*. If we believe that *we* control our own circumstances, we are said to be operating under an internal *locus of control.* Both are always in play and exist in varying ratios in each individual depending on the types of experiences encountered and previous history of reinforcement with them.

Mechanic, mechanical, mechanism – comes from the 14th century Latin *mechanicus* and Greek *mekhanikos* meaning "an engineer." As a noun it can relate to a manual laborer, an artisan, a skilled workman or a pattern of performance. As an adjective it can relate to machine like or automatic actions.

Mediocre, mediocrity – comes from the late 16th century Middle French *mediocre* and Latin *mediocris* meaning "of medium height, moderate or ordinary." It later morphed into the contemporary meaning of "being inferior, unnoticeable or having little value or interest." It can be used as a noun or adjective.

Memory – comes from the 11th century old French *memoire*, 13th century Anglo-French *memorie* and Latin *memoria* meaning "awareness, consciousness, recollection, record and faculty of remembering." In terms of our discussions, it is taking static mental pictures or snapshots of our experiences and storing them in our personal and recallable timeline for future use.

Mind – is the vehicle used for separation (choice) in the domain of *Eros*. The separation is enabled by taking static snapshots of experience and stringing them together forming a perceived timeline. The mind can *only* exist within this timeline. It needs the past, present and future to be able to separate preferences. It is most confounded by our *Intuition*. It is essentially a *dynamic* force but uses *static* information to create its perceived identity through separation and comparison.

Motive, motivation, motif – comes from the 14c Old French *motif* and Medieval Latin *motivus* meaning "moving, impelling." It also relates to "will, drive, something brought forward." The inward movement relative behavior initiated in the early 15th century and its psychological use of "inner or social stimulus for an action" began in 1904.

Observe, observation, observant – comes from the 14th century Old French *observer* meaning to "hold to," as in life conduct and the Latin *observare* meaning "to watch over, look to, attend to, guard from." Its root comes from *ob* meaning "over" + *servare* meaning "to watch or keep safe."

Perceive, perception & perceptual – comes from the 1300s Anglo-French *parceif* and Old Northern French *perceivre* meaning "to notice, see, recognize, understand," and from the Latin *percipere* meaning "to gather, obtain, see entirely, take possession of." Its more contemporary meaning is more figurative and means "to grasp with the mind, learn, comprehend," and is derived from *per* meaning "thoroughly" + *capere* meaning "to grasp, take."

Primary Polarity – is the separation of a newborn's awareness between *Thanatos* and *Eros* upon birth.

Recall, recollection, remember – The earliest meaning originated in the 1580s from the Middle French *rapeler* and *recollection* meaning "to repeal, to gather together again" and the Latin *revocare* and *recollectionem* meaning "to bring back to memory." Remember also comes from the Old French meaning "to recall, bring to mind."

Reflect, reflection, reflex – comes from the 1500s French *reflexion* meaning "to throw back heat or light, refract, deflect" and from the late 14 century Latin *reflectere* and *reflexus* meaning "to bend back, bend backwards, turn away."

Reinforcement - formulates a person's expected responses in life and appears to be dependent on five factors of conditioning: Encouragement, Discouragement and Apathy as paired with consistency or inconsistency.

Resonate, resonant, resonance – comes from the mid 15 century Middle French *resonance* meaning "prolongation of reverberation" and the Latin *resonantia* meaning "echo" and *resonare* meaning "to sound again."

Secondary or Mundane Polarity – is the separation of our tangible world of *Eros* into opposing preferences geared toward our own continuity and survival. As it gains in dominance through increasing tangible worldly experiences, the awareness of *Thanatos* fades into our subconscious and eventually into our unconscious with its effects non-verbally surfacing only when early pre-verbal memories or traumatic experiences are triggered.

Tabula Rasa – comes from the 1530s Latin *tabula rasa* meaning "the mind in its primary state, scraped tablet." Its origins are from *tabula* meaning table + *rasa* or *radere* meaning "to scrape away, erase."

Thanatos – is the urge to return to an undivided sense of oblivion where there are no needs separating us from our total symbiosis with our mother before birth, or perhaps even where we were before our conception. In it exists the field of *intuition,* which is independent of time. It also relates to the 1935 meaning in Freud's psychology, "death instinct." In Geek mythology, Thanatos and Hypnos were the half-brothers in Death and Sleep.

Vibrate, vibration, vibratory – comes from the Latin *vibratis* meaning "to set into tremulous motion, move quickly to and fro, quiver, tremble and shake." Its origins date back 5500 years to the Procto-Indo-European era from *wib-ro* meaning "to turn, vacillate, tremble ecstatically, move quickly to and fro" and the Dutch *wippen* meaning "to swing."

Voluntary, volunteer, volition – comes from the 1600 French *volition,* Middle Latin *volitionem* meaning "will or to wish."

Will – comes from the Old English *willan, wyllan* meaning "to wish, desire, want." It also comes from Old Saxon *willian,* Old Norse *vilja,* Dutch *willen,* German *wollen,* Gothic *wiljan,* Sanskrit *vrnoti,* Latin *volo.* Its earliest known origins are the Procto-Indo-European *wel* and *wol* meaning "to be pleasing."

References & Helpful Reading Material

Adler, Alfred (1927). *Understanding Human Nature: The Psychology of Personality.* One World publications, Oxford, England. ISBN# 978-1-85168-667-4.

Agnes, Michael & Laird, Charles, editors (2002). *Webster's New World Dictionary and Thesaurus.* Hungry Minds, New York, NY. ISBN# 0-7645-6339-4.

Bandler, Richard & Grinder, John (1882). *ReFraming: Neuro-Linguistic Programming and the Transformation of Meaning.* Real People Press, Moab, Ut. ISBN# 0-911226-24-9.

Berne, Eric (1964). *Games People Play: The Basic Handbook of Transactional Analysis.* Ballantine Books, Random House, New York, NY. ISBN# 0-345-41003-3.

Bly, Robert, (1990). *Iron John: A Book About Men.* Addison-West Publishing Company, Inc. New York. ISBN# 0-201-51720-5.

Bradshaw, J. (1988). *Bradshaw On: The Family.* Health Communication Books, Inc., Deerfield Beach, Florida. ISBN# 1-55874-427-4.

Bradshaw, J. (1988). *Healing the Shame that Binds You.* Health Communication Books, Inc., Deerfield Beach, Florida. ISBN# 978-0-7573-0323-4.

Chodron, Pema (1994). *Start from Where You Are: A Guide to Compassionate Living.* Shambala Publishing, Inc. Boston, Mass. ISBN# 1-57062-839-4.

Ekman PhD., Paul, Friesen, Wallace V., (2003). *Unmasking the Face: A Guide to Recognizing Emotions from Facial Expressions.* Malor Books. Cambridge, Ma. ISBN# 1-883536-36-7.

Estes PhD., Clarissa Pinkola, (1992). *Women Who Run With Wolves: Myths and Stories About the Wild Woman Archetype.* Random House Publishing Group. New York. ISBN# 0-345-40987-6.

Firestone, PhD., Robert W. (1985). *The Fantasy Bond: Structure of Defenses.* The Glendon Association, Santa Barbara, Ca. ISBN# 0-9676684-0-9.

Firestone, PhD,. Robert W., Catlett MA, Joyce, (2002). *Conquer Your Critical Inner Voice.* New Harbinger Publications, Inc., Oakland, Ca., ISBN# 1572242876.

Firestone PhD., Robert W., Catlett MA., (2004). *Fear of Intimacy.* American Psychological Association, Washington, DC, ISBN# 1-55798-720-3.

Forward PhD., Susan. (1989). *Toxic Parents: Overcoming Their Harmful Legacy and Reclaiming Your Life.* Random House, New York, N.Y. ISBN# 978-0-553-38140-1.

Forward PhD., Susan. (1997). *Emotional Blackmail.* Harper Collins Publishers, Inc. New York, NY. ISBN# 978-0-06-092897-1.

Fossom, Merle A., Mason, Marilyn J. (1986). *Facing Shame: Families in Recovery.* W.W. Norton & Company. New York, N. Y. ISBN# 0-393-30581-3.

Fritz, R., (1984). *The Path of Least Resistance: Learning to Become the Creative Force in Your Own Life.* Random House. New York, N.Y. ISBN# 0-449-90337-0.

Hallowell M.D., Edward, (2002). *The Childhood Roots of Adult Happiness.* Random House. New York, New York. ISBN# 0-345-44232-6.

Harris, Thomas, (1967). *I'm OK – You're OK.* Harper Collins, New York, N.Y. ISBN# 0-06-072427-7.

Hicks, Esther, Hicks, Jerry. (2009) *The Vortex: Where the Law of Attraction Assembles All Cooperative Relationships.* Hay House, Inc. Carlsbad, California. ISBN# 1-4019-1882-8.

Jeffers PhD., Susan (1987). *Feel the Fear and Do It Anyway.* Fawcett Books/Random House, New York, NY. ISBN# 0-449-90292-7.

Kaufman, G., (1989). *The Psychology of Shame: Theory and Treatment of Shame-Based Syndromes.* New York, New York: Springer Publishing Company. ISBN# 978-082616672-2.

Kelly, Mathew (2005). *Seven Levels of Intimacy.* Simon & Schuster, New York, N.Y., ISBN# 0-7432-6511-4.

Maerz, John L., (2012). *A Mile in Your Shoes: The Road to Self-Actualization Through Compassion.* Lulu Publishing. ISBN# 978-1-105-95262-3.

Maslow, Abraham (1954). *Motivation and Personality.* New York: Harper and Row Publishers. ISBN# 0060419873.

Maslow, A. H. (1943). "A Theory of Human Motivation." Psychological Review, 50, 370-396.

Middleton-Moz, J., (1990). *Shame and Guilt: Masters of Disguise.* Health Communications, Inc., Deerfield Beach, Florida. ISBN# 978-1-558874-072-3,.

Miller, Alice, (2002). *For Your Own Good: Hidden Cruelty in Child-Rearing and the Roots of Violence.* Farrar, Straus & Giroux, Frankfurt, Germany. ISBN# 0-374-52269-3.

Morrison, Andrew P. (1997). *Shame: The Underside of Narcissism.* The Analytic Press. ISBN# 0881-632-805.

Onions, C.T., Friedrichsen, G.W.S., Burchfield, R.W, editors (1966). *The Oxford Dictionary of English Etymology.* Oxford University Press, New York. ISBN# 978-0-19-86112-7.

Peck M.D., Scott, (1978). *The Road Less Traveled.* Simon & Schuster, New York, New York. ISBN# 0-684-84724-8.

Rand, Ayn, (1961). *The Virtue of Selfishness.* The Penguin Group (USA) Inc., New York, New York. ISBN# 978-0-451-16393-6

Reber, A., Allen, R., & Reber, E., (1985). *Penguin Dictionary of Psychology.* Penguin Books, Ltd., London, England. ISBN# 978-0-141-03024-1.

Robbins, Anthony, (1986). *Unlimited Power.* A Fireside Book Published by Simon & Schuster. New york, N.Y. ISBN# 0-684-84577-6.

Rosenblatt, F., Farrow, J.T, Herblin, W.F. *"Transfer of conditioned responses from trained rats to untrained rats by means of a brain extract."* <u>Nature.</u> 1966 Jan 1;209(5018):46-8. PMID: 5925330

Ruumet, Hillevi, PhD., (2006). *Pathways of the Soul: Exploring the Human Journey.* Trafford Pub., Victoria, BC, Canada. ISBN# 1412-092-361.

Scheff, T. J., (1995). "Shame and Related Emotions: An Overview." The American Behavioral Scientist, 38, 1053-1059.

Seligman, M.E.P. (1975). *Helplessness: On Depression, Development, and Death.* W.H. Freeman. San Francisco, Calif. ISBN# 0-7167-2328-X.

Seligman, M.E.P., Maier, Steven F., Peterson, Christopher, (1993). *Learned Helplessness: A Theory for the Age of Control.* Oxford university Press. New York, N.Y. ISBN# 0-19-504467-3.

Watts, Alan, (1966). *The Book: On the Taboo Against Knowing Who You Are.* Vintage Books, Random House, Inc., New York, N.Y. ISBN# 0-679-723000-5.

Watts, Alan, (1951). *The Wisdom of Insecurity.* Pantheon Books, Random House, Inc., New York, N.Y. ISBN# 0-394-70468-1.

...About the Author

J. LAWRENCE MAERZ, B.A.

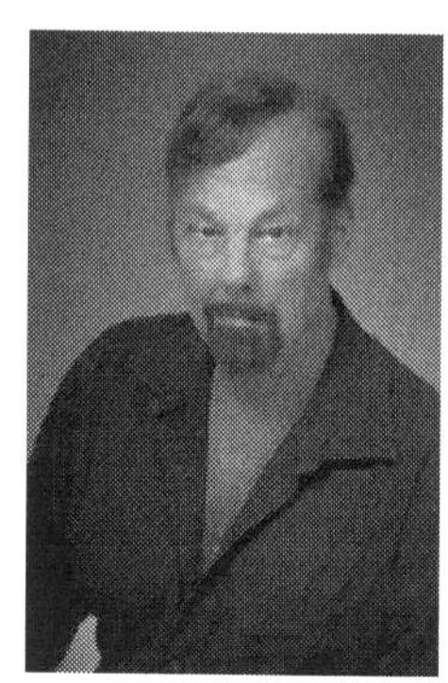

I'm an author, professional speaker and coach with a specialization in psychological study. Having worked as a counselor and as a case manager with teen substance abuse and in social services in child protection I'm a seasoned personal coach, adviser and lecturer and have a diverse background in the human potentials field incorporating personality influences, shadow work, nutritional needs, creative expression and personal desires while uncovering innate abilities and hidden potentials for my clients. I'm dedicated toward raising awareness and share my own unique understandings and perspectives about life's journey and meaning. I, also, recognize the need for balance and accountability on our mental, physical and emotional levels as well as fulfilling our spiritual potential through our individual experiences.

I've published five books including this one. The most recent is entitled "*A MILE IN YOUR SHOES: The Road to Actualization Through Compassion*" which covers the origins and effects of shame based child-rearing practices while offering techniques to overcome the resulting feelings of inferiority without the assistance of a therapist. You can find my most current work available at:

www.JohnMaerz.com

www.AwakeandThinking.com

ELEMENTARY FEELINGS

Happiness
Sadness
Anger
Disgust
Surprise
Fear
Apathy

EMOTIONS

Abandoned	Denounced
Abused	Depressed
Amused	Deserted
Annoyed	Destitute
Appreciated	Diminished
Appreciative	Disappointed
Ashamed	Discouraged
Awestruck	Doubtful
Beaten	Eager
Blissful	Edged Out
Blocked	Embarrassed
Bored	Empowered
Burned Out	Empty
Childish	Enabled
Compressed	Energized
Content	Enraged
Denied	Enthralled

Enthusiastic

Exhausted

Excited

Excommunicated

Fooled

Free

Frustrated

Grief Stricken

Guilty

Hateful

Healthy

Hopeful

Hopeless

Hurt

Ignored

Impatient

Immature

Important

Infuriated

Invalidated

Irritated

Jealous

Joyful

Lonely

Lost

Manipulated

Misplaced

Mortified

Nurtured

Oppressed

Optimistic

Ostracized

Out of Place

Overjoyed

Overstressed

Over-stimulated

Overwhelmed

Passionate

Played

Powerful

Powerless

Protected

Punished

Raped

Rebuked

Redeemed

Resentful

Ridiculous

Refused

Regenerated

Rejected

Removed

Renewed

Restored

Singled Out

Small

Stupid

Superfluous

Suppressed

Ugly

Unappreciated

Unbalanced

Uncomfortable

Undesirable

Ungrateful

Unhealthy

Unimportant
Unlovable
Unnatural
Unnecessary
Unwanted
Unwelcome
Unworthy
Useless

Validated
Vengeful
Venomous
Vindicated
Weird
Welcome
Worried

ACTIONS

Abuse
Antagonize
Burn
Caress
Combat
Compliment
Congratulate
Contend
Cry
Denigrate
Deny
Destroy
Die
Disappear
Drown
Educate
Escape
Excommunicate
Expel
Explode
Fondle
Hide

Hit
Hold
Hug
Hurt
Ignore
Imprison
Insult
Kill
Kiss
Laugh
Lay
Leave
Mash
Melt
Murder
Obliterate
Ostracize
Poke
Push
Punch
Punish
Rape

Refuse
Remove
Run
Scold
Scream
Shrink

Slap
Spank
Stop
Strip
Tell
Tickl

JUDGMENTS

Abusive
Amusing
Antagonistic
Beautiful
Brash
Cheap
Chivalrous
Combative
Contentious
Corrupt
Creepy
Crooked
Crude Despicable
Devious
Discourteous
Disgusting
Dishonest
Educated
Egotistical
Evil
Fastidious
Fat
Filthy

Foolish
Generous
Holy
Honest
Humble
Ignorant
Illiterate
Impractical
Irreverent
Lazy
Loud
Lovely
Loving
Neat
Ornery
Overbearing
Practical
Retarded
Resentful
Ridiculous
Retiring
Rude
Sacred

Silly
Skinny
Slippery
Sloppy
Smart
Smelly
Studious

Superfluous
Stupid
Ugly
Uneducated
Useless
Waste

For the "PEOPLE" fill in, please name the person or their position in your life who best fits each of the 6 categories. You may fill in more than one for each but make sure the best fit appears first. For the Emotional Trail fill in, make six copies, one each for the "PEOPLE" you listed, then fill in the blanks relative to each person. I've included a list of most of the words that I can think of but you may think of more. Follow the key on the bottom of the form to know which choices from which group to fill in for each blank: **F**=Elementary Feeling, **E**=Emotion, **A**=Action or **J**=Judgment. **Make sure that #7 is an Elementary Feeling only.**

PEOPLE

1) The most important person in my life is______________________.

2) The most unimportant person in my life is______________.

3) The person I love the most is______________________________.

4) The person I dislike or hate the most is______________.

5) The person I envy the most is ______________________.

6) The person I fear the most is______________________________.

EMOTIONAL TRAIL

1) The person I (F or E) ______________the most is (F or E) ______________.

2) When I think about them I am (F or E) ______________.

3) Feeling (F or E) ______________ this about them makes me want to (A) ___________.

4) When I imagine myself doing this I feel (F or E) _______________.

5) When I feel (F or E)_____________________I know that I am being
   (J)_______________

6) Being (J) ______________I feel (F or E) __________ and I want to
   (A)_________________________

7) This only makes me feel (F only) ________________________ .

8) Why do you think this makes you feel as you do in question #7

   ____
   ____.

*Ledger Key: F = Feeling, E = Emotion, A = Action, J =
Judgment*

MOTIVATIONAL ASSESSMENT

(Who Makes the Rules for You?)

1) What is it in you that needs to remain hidden so you won't feel embarrassed, exposed, out of control or diminished?

2) To whom have you assigned the duty of determining your value? Do you have to keep your mate happy and safe? Must you work at not disappointing your parents? Will your best friend crumble if you're not there for them? Will no one do the job if you don't? Will they not survive if you're not there to care for them?

3) If you don't "live up" to the duty, what will you lose?

4) What image do you feel that you must maintain in order to remain in the "good graces" of the people who are important to you?

5) What famous figure is it that you'd like to be like? Why?

6) List at least five people you feel responsible to and for and name the responsibility for each.

7) What part does religion play in your life? Where does your belief emanate from?

8) Whom is it that will give you the best reflection of how you're coming across to others and why do you trust *them* more than anyone else?

9) Who is it that best accepts you for who you are? What are they able to accept and overlook in you? (be specific)

10) What would your best friend say about your character?

11) What would your worst enemy say about your character?

12) What do you do well in spite of what others may say or think about you?

13) What makes this possible?

14) How do you know when you're not living up to *your* potential?